FAMILY

PREPARING FOR BABY

FAMILY MATTERS

PREPARING FOR BABY

ROS MEEK

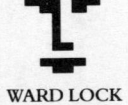

WARD LOCK

Acknowledgement
This book is dedicated to my husband Graham, father of Emily, William and Jessica. Together we have laughed, cried and agonized over parenthood — but it has been worth it!

Also to my girl-friends with whom I have shared the ups-and-downs of pregnancy, childbirth and children. Nothing can replace the many sanity-saving evenings that we have spent together.

First published in 1990 by Ward Lock
Villiers House, 41/47 Strand, London WC2N 5JE, England

A Cassell imprint

© Ward Lock Limited 1990

All rights reserved. No part of this publication
may be reproduced or transmitted in any form or
by any means, electronic or mechanical including
photocopying, recording or any information storage
or retrieval system, without prior permission
in writing from the publishers.

Changing bag pattern reproduced by kind permission of *Mother Magazine*.

Dungaree pattern reproduced from *The Royal Baby: Nursery and Furnishing Handbook* by Sue James, published by Orbis.

Knits for baby reproduced from *Nursery Rhyme Knits* by Sue Locke, published by Ward Lock.

British Library Cataloguing in Publication Data
Meek, Ros
  Preparing for baby. — (Family matters)
  1. Parenthood. Personal adjustment
  I. Title
  306.8'74

ISBN 0–7063–6883–5

Text filmset by Columns of Reading

Printed and bound in Great Britain by Collins

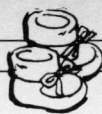

CONTENTS

INTRODUCTION	**7**
Preconception	8
Alcohol	10
Smoking	10
Medicines and Pills	11
At Work	12
Miscarriage	13
ARE YOU — AREN'T YOU PREGNANT?	**15**
Am I Pregnant?	15
Who Can I Tell?	18
Ideas	19
YOUR PREGNANCY CONFIRMED	**20**
The Ante-natal Clinic	22
EXERCISING IN PREGNANCY	**26**
Look after your back	28
PREGNANCY WORRIES	**30**
Prevention of Problems	30
Relaxation	31
Pregnancy Problems	32
YOUR DEVELOPING BABY	**40**

CONTENTS

DESIGNS TO KNIT OR SEW — 47

MAKING YOUR HOME READY — 63
Preparing the Baby's Room — 64
Advantages and Disadvantages of Baby being in your Room — 65

WHAT YOU NEED FOR YOUR BABY — 72
Essential Items of Equipment — 75
Social Security Benefits — 75
Complaint Procedure — 76
Buying Second-hand — 76

MUM'S ESSENTIALS — 78
Getting Ready for Birth — 82

PREPARING FOR LABOUR — 85
What is Labour? — 85
Suggestions for your Birth Plan — 86

USEFUL ORGANIZATIONS AND FURTHER INFORMATION — 88

INDEX — 93

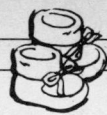

INTRODUCTION

There are several reasons why you may have decided to buy this book. It may be that you are thinking about having a baby some time in the near future and want to know what you can do to prepare yourself for this exciting event. Perhaps you have just found out that you are pregnant or you are looking for information about how to tell if you are expecting a baby. Whatever your reason, you will find some answers here together with information to allow you and your partner to make informed choices about your pregnancy.

Attitudes to pregnant women have changed considerably during the past 20 years largely due to pressure from women themselves who resented the lack of freedom and choice in pregnancy and childbirth. Support groups, such as the National Childbirth Trust, were formed to demand accurate detailed information for women in the ante-natal clinics and labour wards *and to lobby for increased consumer participation*. The medical profession was seen as having taken over and mechanized the natural process of pregnancy and labour. No longer were the 'hands-on' skills of the friendly midwife valued; the medical profession preferred the certainty of ultrasound scans, monitoring, artificially induced labours and epidurals and episiotomies to 'ease' the labour. All these 'high tech' skills have their place, of course, and should not be undervalued, but in the 1970s the practice of listening to women was forgotten largely to make way for more

INTRODUCTION

convenient daytime births for the medical profession.

Thankfully the medical profession and particularly midwives have now listened and taken action on behalf of pregnant women.

So what are the changes that you might expect to find? Firstly you will be given lots of information, by doctors, midwives and commercial companies all seeking to help you through this 'natural process'. Having been given this information you will be encouraged to ask questions about your case and share any worries you may have. Partners are seen by most hospitals now as an essential part of the process of pregnancy and will be welcomed at ante-natal clinics, ultrasound scans, preparation for parenthood groups and in the labour ward. If you don't have a partner then a friend, sister or mother will be just as welcome.

Sometimes with all the things that need to be thought about and acted upon, you may become confused or anxious. Talk to other women who are pregnant or who have had children; they will understand and give you support. This book will help you to get things into perspective, and to look to the future months with anticipation and confidence. Your GP, midwife and health visitor will also be available for you to discuss things with. You will doubtless find that there are many other self-styled experts who will give you advice, warn of so-called dangers and tell you old wives' tales. The secret is to nod wisely and check it out for yourself!

PRECONCEPTION

The idea of preconceptual care, that is thinking about your state of health *before* you try to become pregnant, is something that has gained in popularity as more has become known about conception and the complex interaction between mother and baby in the womb.

One of the most significant facts that has come to light

INTRODUCTION

is that the mother's nutritional state on becoming pregnant will influence the baby's birth weight and chances of survival. Overweight women have a slightly increased risk of problems in early and late pregnancy. Because of this, it is advisable that severely overweight women should try to lose weight in advance of becoming pregnant. It is important to remember that it is dangerous to go on a crash diet as soon as you know that you are pregnant because essential nutrient stores may become depleted.

Malnutrition can reduce fertility and deprive the unborn baby of essential nutrients, so it is important that women achieve a suitable weight before becoming pregnant. The foetus is at its most vulnerable nutritionally in the few weeks following conception. A varied diet will be more likely to ensure an adequate intake of all nutrients.

Some medical research has shown that taking multi-vitamins, particularly folic acid, reduces the risk of spina bifida. At present, however, the advice is that unless you are at risk of anaemia then folic acid supplements are not necessary. If vitamins are advised they should be started at least 28 days before conception so that high enough blood levels can be reached.

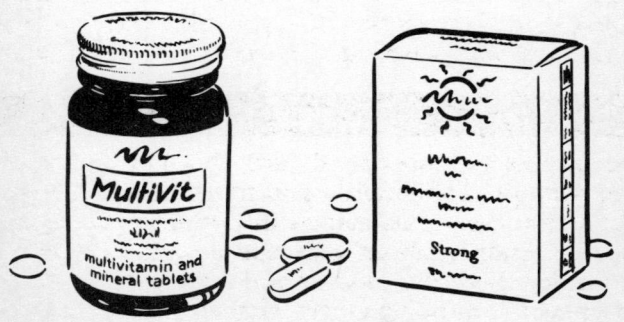

ALCOHOL

This is best avoided by those wishing to become pregnant because it affects the absorption of several different nutrients into the bloodstream. It also affects the removal rate from the body. Once pregnant the occasional drink is less likely to cause harm, though over two units of alcohol daily (two glasses of wine) has been shown to result in lower birthweight babies. Alcohol also affects male fertility. It would seem a sensible precaution, therefore, to reduce alcohol consumption before pregnancy and preferably to cut it out to reduce any risk. If you drink a lot of alcohol and feel that you will have problems giving it up, contact Alcohol Concern (see page 88). It will send you advice and information about local help for women.

SMOKING

It harms both you and your developing baby. It can restrict the baby's growth and cause premature delivery or miscarriage. So is it worth it?

I need to smoke so I can relax —
Nicotine makes your baby's heart beat too fast.

It helps me to stop putting on weight —
Sensible eating will do this, too, without harming your unborn child

I'll have a smaller baby and therefore an easier labour if I smoke —
The carbon monoxide in the cigarette will pass into your baby's bloodstream depriving your baby of some oxygen and therefore stopping it from growing as fast as it needs to.

Smoking stops me worrying about things —
No one is saying that it is easy to give up smoking. Try to persuade your partner or a friend to give up with you.

Don't reach for a cigarette ...

☆ 1. Put something else in your hands — try knitting, sewing, crochet. Join a local class if you don't know how to.

☆ 2. Doodling or carrying worry beads can help.

☆ 3. When you feel the urge, do something else — eat an apple, drink some water, try some deep breathing.

☆ 4. Swimming is good for relaxing and will also increase your lung capacity and help you feel good about giving up smoking.

Give yourself something to aim for, perhaps a new dress, a facial or a night at the theatre. You will have saved up the money in no time at all, so fix a date and stick to it. Avoid pubs, top decks of buses and places where others smoke. Contact ASH. It will send you useful information (see page 88). If you can't give up, then cut down drastically and make sure that you are eating a well-balanced diet.

MEDICINES AND PILLS

Many medicines and pills, even those that are bought without prescriptions, can cause harm to a developing baby. It is, therefore, best to avoid taking any medicines whilst you are trying to have a baby. If you need to take tablets regularly for a condition, such as diabetes or high blood pressure, have a chat with your doctor first and tell him that you want to become pregnant. He will know which tablets are safest during pregnancy. If you are given a prescription during pregnancy, remind your doctor and ask your pharmacist about anything that you want to buy in the chemist shop.

Drugs can seriously affect your developing baby and can even mean that your baby could be born dependent on drugs. If you need help about coming off drugs ring SCODA (Standing Conference on Drug Abuse) and ask for information about local groups (see page 90).

AT WORK

Some work that is done in industry can be potentially harmful to a baby especially in the early weeks. Work that is particularly physical, or tiring, or involves exposure to chemicals, metals or radiation can cause infertility. If you think you might be at risk, speak to the Personnel Department or your trade union. They will treat your discussion in confidence. If necessary you can obtain a written assurance from your employer that there is no harm in you continuing to do your job.

If your job does put you at risk, ask to be moved to another area, provided with protective clothing or avoid the specific area where there is risk. If there is no alternative job available then you may have to leave or be dismissed from employment. It is better to be aware of this situation before becoming pregnant, so make an appointment to see your Union Representative or Personnel Manager.

If you feel you would like to have more information about preparing yourself for pregnancy, ask your GP, Family Planning Clinic or local community health council if there is a preconceptual care clinic in the area. Remember, however, that it is not an insurance policy for immediate conception or indeed for a perfect baby, though it does cut down some of the risks. If you have any inherited abnormalities in your family, such as cystic fibrosis or Down's syndrome, you can be referred by your GP to a genetic counsellor who will be able to tell you what the risks are.

If you do not become pregnant straight away try not to worry. Anxiety can make conception more difficult and one in five couples take up to a year to conceive. If you have been trying for over a year, seek help from your GP. See pages 88–89 for further information on BPAS and National Association for the Childless.

MISCARRIAGE

A small proportion of women suffer miscarriage in early pregnancy. It is a sad fact that one in ten pregnancies end this way. In the past it was regarded as nature's way of removing a pregnancy that had gone wrong and often women were not even aware that they were pregnant. Today with the control of fertility being seen largely as a woman's responsibility (whether we like it or not) the knowledge of being pregnant comes earlier and can be confirmed earlier.

Whenever miscarriage happens it is a terrible shock. First you may feel anger and grief which may give way to the worry about whether you will be able to have a baby. You may find that talking to other women, especially those who have had miscarriages themselves, is helpful. The Miscarriage Association (see page 91) is a group which will counsel you and share your concerns.

Miscarriage sometimes follows bleeding in early pregnancy, so if you start to bleed sit down and rest, particularly if you are experiencing any pain. It is best to speak to your GP if the bleeding continues and you should avoid sex for a couple of weeks. Some women have an 'implantation bleed' which happens when the egg starts to embed itself in the uterus. This is not a sign of a miscarriage, though it is best to mention it to the doctor as it will help to determine the end of your pregnancy.

Miscarriages which happen after the first three months of pregnancy are more rare and are often caused by what doctors call an 'incompetent cervix'. This means that the cervix or neck of the womb is not remaining closed. It may have been weakened by a previous birth or a D and C. In these cases a Shirodkar suture or stitch can keep the cervix closed.

MISCARRIAGE

Any bleeding in pregnancy should be mentioned to your doctor or midwife.

If you do bleed, try to remember:

- How much bleeding there was
- Whether it was fresh red blood or brownish
- Whether the blood was clotted or jellylike
- What you were doing at the time
- Whether you had pain with the bleeding.

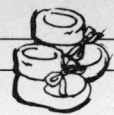

ARE YOU — AREN'T YOU PREGNANT?

Not everyone will know immediately they become pregnant. Some women even come to hospital in labour not having realized they were pregnant — but that is very rare thankfully! Once you have decided that you want to have a baby it will help if you keep a diary of your periods. The date that your baby will be due can then be accurately worked out.

AM I PREGNANT?

- Do you feel sick in the morning or during the day?
- Have your breasts become fuller and more sensitive?
- Do you need to get up to go to the lavatory at night?
- Do you feel tired, especially after meals?
- Have you gone off some foods or have a metallic taste in your mouth?
- Do you have more vaginal discharge than usual?
- Are you constipated when it is not normally a problem?

If you have some of these symptoms and you have missed your period you can make an appointment to see your doctor for a pregnancy test. Pregnancy tests can also be bought from the chemist or can be done for you by your GP, at the Family Planning Clinic or by a

January	1	2	3	4	5	6	7	8	9	10	11	12	13	14	15	16	17	18	19	20	21	22	23	24	25	26	27	28	29	30	31	January
October	8	9	10	11	12	13	14	15	16	17	18	19	20	21	22	23	24	25	26	27	28	29	30	31	1	2	3	4	5	6	7	November
February	**1**	**2**	**3**	**4**	**5**	**6**	**7**	**8**	**9**	**10**	**11**	**12**	**13**	**14**	**15**	**16**	**17**	**18**	**19**	**20**	**21**	**22**	**23**	**24**	**25**	**26**	**27**	**28**				**February**
November	8	9	10	11	12	13	14	15	16	17	18	19	20	21	22	23	24	25	26	27	28	29	30	1	2	3	4	5				December
March	**1**	**2**	**3**	**4**	**5**	**6**	**7**	**8**	**9**	**10**	**11**	**12**	**13**	**14**	**15**	**16**	**17**	**18**	**19**	**20**	**21**	**22**	**23**	**24**	**25**	**26**	**27**	**28**	**29**	**30**	**31**	**March**
December	6	7	8	9	10	11	12	13	14	15	16	17	18	19	20	21	22	23	24	25	26	27	28	29	30	31	1	2	3	4	5	January
April	**1**	**2**	**3**	**4**	**5**	**6**	**7**	**8**	**9**	**10**	**11**	**12**	**13**	**14**	**15**	**16**	**17**	**18**	**19**	**20**	**21**	**22**	**23**	**24**	**25**	**26**	**27**	**28**	**29**	**30**		**April**
January	6	7	8	9	10	11	12	13	14	15	16	17	18	19	20	21	22	23	24	25	26	27	28	29	30	31	1	2	3	4		February
May	**1**	**2**	**3**	**4**	**5**	**6**	**7**	**8**	**9**	**10**	**11**	**12**	**13**	**14**	**15**	**16**	**17**	**18**	**19**	**20**	**21**	**22**	**23**	**24**	**25**	**26**	**27**	**28**	**29**	**30**	**31**	**May**
February	5	6	7	8	9	10	11	12	13	14	15	16	17	18	19	20	21	22	23	24	25	26	27	28	1	2	3	4	5	6	7	March
June	**1**	**2**	**3**	**4**	**5**	**6**	**7**	**8**	**9**	**10**	**11**	**12**	**13**	**14**	**15**	**16**	**17**	**18**	**19**	**20**	**21**	**22**	**23**	**24**	**25**	**26**	**27**	**28**	**29**	**30**		**June**
March	8	9	10	11	12	13	14	15	16	17	18	19	20	21	22	23	24	25	26	27	28	29	30	31	1	2	3	4	5	6		April
July	**1**	**2**	**3**	**4**	**5**	**6**	**7**	**8**	**9**	**10**	**11**	**12**	**13**	**14**	**15**	**16**	**17**	**18**	**19**	**20**	**21**	**22**	**23**	**24**	**25**	**26**	**27**	**28**	**29**	**30**	**31**	**July**
April	7	8	9	10	11	12	13	14	15	16	17	18	19	20	21	22	23	24	25	26	27	28	29	30	1	2	3	4	5	6	7	May
August	**1**	**2**	**3**	**4**	**5**	**6**	**7**	**8**	**9**	**10**	**11**	**12**	**13**	**14**	**15**	**16**	**17**	**18**	**19**	**20**	**21**	**22**	**23**	**24**	**25**	**26**	**27**	**28**	**29**	**30**	**31**	**August**
May	8	9	10	11	12	13	14	15	16	17	18	19	20	21	22	23	24	25	26	27	28	29	30	31	1	2	3	4	5	6	7	June
September	**1**	**2**	**3**	**4**	**5**	**6**	**7**	**8**	**9**	**10**	**11**	**12**	**13**	**14**	**15**	**16**	**17**	**18**	**19**	**20**	**21**	**22**	**23**	**24**	**25**	**26**	**27**	**28**	**29**	**30**		**September**
June	8	9	10	11	12	13	14	15	16	17	18	19	20	21	22	23	24	25	26	27	28	29	30	1	2	3	4	5	6	7		July
October	**1**	**2**	**3**	**4**	**5**	**6**	**7**	**8**	**9**	**10**	**11**	**12**	**13**	**14**	**15**	**16**	**17**	**18**	**19**	**20**	**21**	**22**	**23**	**24**	**25**	**26**	**27**	**28**	**29**	**30**	**31**	**October**
July	8	9	10	11	12	13	14	15	16	17	18	19	20	21	22	23	24	25	26	27	28	29	30	31	1	2	3	4	5	6	7	August
November	**1**	**2**	**3**	**4**	**5**	**6**	**7**	**8**	**9**	**10**	**11**	**12**	**13**	**14**	**15**	**16**	**17**	**18**	**19**	**20**	**21**	**22**	**23**	**24**	**25**	**26**	**27**	**28**	**29**	**30**		**November**
August	8	9	10	11	12	13	14	15	16	17	18	19	20	21	22	23	24	25	26	27	28	29	30	31	1	2	3	4	5	6		September
December	**1**	**2**	**3**	**4**	**5**	**6**	**7**	**8**	**9**	**10**	**11**	**12**	**13**	**14**	**15**	**16**	**17**	**18**	**19**	**20**	**21**	**22**	**23**	**24**	**25**	**26**	**27**	**28**	**29**	**30**	**31**	**December**
September	7	8	9	10	11	12	13	14	15	16	17	18	19	20	21	22	23	24	25	26	27	28	29	30	1	2	3	4	5	6	7	October

Pick out the date of the first day of your last monthly period from the figures in black. The date your baby is due is immediately underneath.

AM I PREGNANT?

chemist. Some other clinics also offer these services for a small fee. Do-it-yourself kits are now very reliable provided you follow the instructions, but can be quite expensive.

Once you have had a positive result, you can make an appointment to see your GP so that you can start to think about your ante-natal care and where to have your baby. Your GP will also confirm when your baby is due. This is known as the EDD (estimated date of delivery). You can work it out for yourself using this chart.

So now you have had your pregnancy confirmed — you really are expecting a baby — how do you feel?

☆ Ecstatic
☆ Happy
☆ Nothing special
☆ Uncertain
☆ Apprehensive
☆ Trapped
☆ Frightened

Women feel all these emotions so do not feel worried if you don't feel how you imagined. For a start, you may feel very tired and out of sorts. Your body is starting to change as the pregnancy hormones take over.

WHO CAN I TELL?

Some women want to tell everyone straight away but others are more cautious, particularly if they have had previous miscarriages. It is up to you when you tell people. It is rather a nice secret to keep to yourself for a day or so — some find it quite hard to tell their partner. By not telling everyone you will give yourself a little more time to adjust.

Some men feel particularly apprehensive once the news is confirmed. Even when they are desperately keen, the fear of future responsibilities can weigh heavily. Try to talk together about your feelings. Pregnancy is a time for sharing and caring.

As soon as you realize that you are pregnant you will notice lots of other pregnant women and those with babies; you will look in prams and gaze into baby-shop windows — a whole new world is opening up for you.

Most women want to find out as much as they can about pregnancy and childbirth. Where can you find out more?

Mother and
Mother-in-law

Telephone Help lines

Other mums

Preparation for Parenthood groups

Books (see pages 91–92)

Health professionals:
GP, midwife, health visitor

Magazines (see page 91)

TV programmes

Videos (see page 92)

The earlier you see your GP and make your first appointment at the booking-in clinic, the sooner you will feel part of the 'club'. Motherhood does seem to be a sort of club that you are admitted to once you have been through the ritual of childbirth.

IDEAS

☆ Why not have a pregnancy notebook? It will be fun to look back on once you have had the baby and interesting to look at should you decide to have another.
☆ Start with a page about yourself, your height, weight and so on. Perhaps a photograph?
☆ Write down how you found out you were pregnant and what you feel about it. Try to remember people's reactions and their predictions as to your baby's sex.
☆ Think about what seems important to you about pregacy and the weeks ahead.
☆ Jot down any dreams you may have.

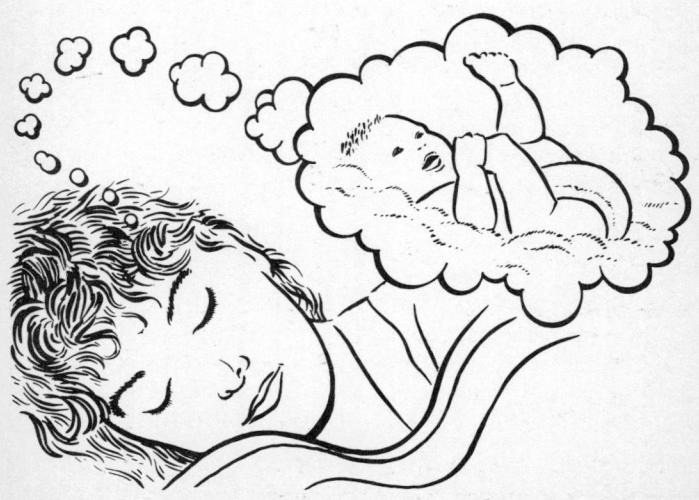

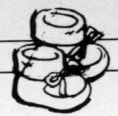

YOUR PREGNANCY CONFIRMED

Once your pregnancy is confirmed your GP will tell you about the local facilities for ante-natal care and you can discuss where you would like to have your baby. What are the options?

★ ***SHARED CARE*** This is when you go to your GP for most of your ante-natal appointments, where you will be seen by the Practice Midwife or one of the GPs. Occasionally you will be asked to go to the hospital for an ultrasound scan or for a check-up, particularly at the end of the pregnancy.

★ ***FULL HOSPITAL CARE*** Not all GPs offer shared care so, in this case, you will go to the hospital for all your appointments.

★ ***DOMINO CARE*** This is where you have your baby in a GP unit or at home. You will mainly be looked after by the GP and Community Midwives.

★ ***HOME BIRTH*** The medical profession in general feels that the safest place for you to have your baby is in a hospital, where everything is on hand if it should be needed. However, this may not be how you would like to have your baby, and, if all goes well, you may prefer to stay in your own home with a midwife.

In general, a home birth if it is planned well in advance, is safe for a healthy woman. You may meet opposition to your wishes to have a home delivery, and it may be necessary for you to change your GP if he does not do home deliveries. You may also consider contacting an Independent Midwife.

If you decide to have your baby at home you may well feel more in control of the situation and therefore require less pain relief. Gas and air, and pethidine, can be given to ease the pain, but epidurals cannot be given.

If during the labour the GP or midwife feels that you need to have a Caesarean section to delivery the baby you may have to go into hospital. If your labour is very lengthy, or if you bleed heavily afterwards, it may also be necessary to transfer you to hospital. Your baby's condition may also mean that you could be transferred, particularly if there are problems with the heart rate or breathing.

If you are undecided about where to have your baby, try to talk to other women in your area who have had home deliveries. They will be a mine of information. Sheila Kitzinger's book *Birth at Home* (see page 91) is also full of valuable information.

If you have chosen a hospital birth your GP will give you a booking letter to take to the hospital. Once the hospital has the letter it will ask you to come to the Ante-natal Booking Clinic. Most women go to the Clinic between 9 and 14 weeks of pregnancy to meet the hospital staff and be booked into the hospital system.

THE ANTE-NATAL CLINIC

It is helpful to talk to other mums about your local clinic. There are often some tips that others have found helpful and this may make your first visit easier. Try to write down any questions for the midwife or doctor because, in the hustle–and–bustle, you may forget something that has been bothering you. The golden rule in pregnancy is *don't leave questions unanswered*. You are not ill and should not be treated as such. You are entitled to information and answers to your questions. You need to feel in control. However approachable the doctor might be the relationship between doctor and pregnant woman is often unequal. Try to remember that pregnancy is a time when you should feel good and assertive about yourself and your growing baby. The more communicative you are with the healthcare professionals, the more your self-confidence will grow.

Here are some questions that you may want answered:
☆ How often will I come to the Clinic?
☆ What tests are performed, and when and why?
☆ Are ante-natal classes held at the hospital?
☆ Can I see round the wards before I am admitted?
☆ Is there a special care baby unit at the hospital?
☆ Do you have facilities for 'natural' birth?
☆ How long will I stay in hospital after the birth?
☆ Who can visit me in hospital?

A midwife will want to talk to you about you and your family's medical history and tell you about the hospital and your care. You can talk about where and how you want to have your baby.

Another part of your 'booking visit' is the tests and examination by the doctor, though in some areas it is performed by a midwife. To guide you through this examination, here are the usual tests that you can expect.

THE ANTE-NATAL CLINIC

* **BLOOD TEST** — To find out your blood group. To measure the haemoglobin (iron level). To check for sexually–transmitted diseases, so they can be treated quickly.

* **BREASTS EXAMINED** — To detect inverted nipples.

* **TUMMY EXAMINED** — To check the size of uterus and compare this with the date of your last period.

* **INTERNAL EXAMINATION** — Not all doctors do an internal examination. A swab may be taken if an infection is suspected. A cervical smear will be done.

* **BLOOD PRESSURE** — To check and record your early pregnancy level, so that any subsequent rise can be identified.

You will also have your weight checked and urine tested at each visit. The urine is checked to make sure that there is no infection and also to check for the presence of sugar which may indicate that you are diabetic.

If you are worried about HIV (Aids) you can discuss this confidentially with your midwife or doctor.

At the end of your visit you will be given a co-operation card (co-op card) which will record your visits to the GP or hospital. Carry it with you all the time so that if you are ill away from home, all your details will be at hand. It also has your GP, midwife and hospital's telephone number on it. If you do not understand the notes, please ask!

The Ante-natal Clinic is not always the most welcoming of places, but hospitals are gradually waking up to the fact that if they make them more friendly, more people will come and everyone will be less tense.

THE ANTE-NATAL CLINIC

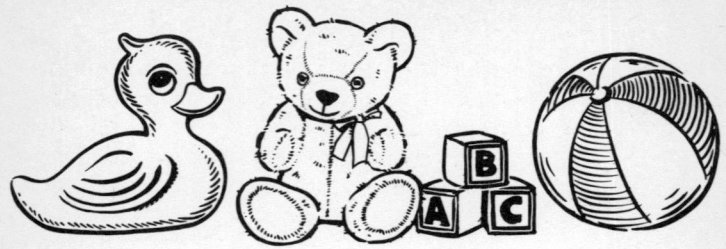

You can use these visits to:

☆ Chat to other women about how they are experiencing their pregnancy.
☆ Find out about local facilities like mother–and–baby clubs, baby feeding and changing rooms, cheap shops for babywear and equipment.
☆ Watch videos on health-related subjects.
☆ *Sit* and think about you for a change!

Some hospitals have crèche facilities so that other children can be cared for while you wait.

If you feel that the Ante-natal Clinic is not as welcoming as it might be, or if there is a specific problem, speak to the Sister in charge. If you are reluctant to do this, you can write to your local Community Health Council, or contact your local branch of the National Childbirth Trust (see page 89).

You will be asked to visit your Ante-natal Clinic or GP every four weeks until you are 28 weeks pregnant. After this it will be every two weeks until 36 weeks and weekly from then on.

You are entitled to time off from work to attend the Ante-natal Clinic. You are also entitled to certain benefits depending on your circumstances. Leaflet FB8, which is available from Post Offices or DHSS offices, will help. Social Workers are also available at the hospital. If you have any worries, ask to speak to one when you next visit the clinic.

What you might be entitled to:

☆ Statutory maternity pay — for women in employment.
☆ Maternity allowance — for those who have recently ceased employment.
☆ Free dental treatment until your child is one year old.
☆ Free chiropody if you have a problem with your feet.

For advice on these benefits you can also phone Freeline Social Security 0800–666555 or Maternity Alliance (see page 89).

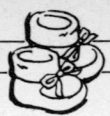

EXERCISE IN PREGNANCY

Most of us would agree that we don't take enough physical exercise, even though we may be on the go all day. In pregnancy a good level of regular exercise is very beneficial.

> **Why should I exercise?**
> ☆ Exercise makes you feel good — after you have done it! It tones up your muscles to cope with your growing pregnancy and labour.
> ☆ Exercise helps you regain your pre-pregnancy shape more easily after the birth of your baby.
> ☆ Exercise improves the blood circulation in your body which, in turn, sends more blood to your developing baby.
> ☆ Exercise relaxes your body and relieves tension. This means it helps you to sleep at night and gives you a general feeling of well-being.

It is up to you to be sensible about what kind of exercise you undertake and for what duration. After all, you are the best judge of what makes you feel good and what appears to be a strain. Try to aim for a combination of rest and exercise. This will vary from perhaps very

EXERCISE IN PREGNANCY

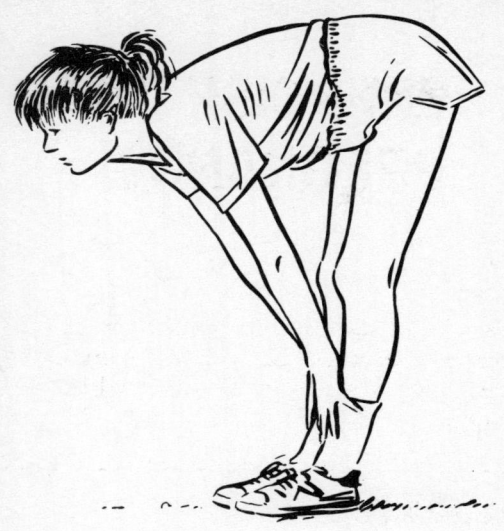

little in the early weeks, a very active spell in the middle of pregnancy and a general slowing up or change of exercise as you prepare for labour.

Helpful points to bear in mind
☆ If you are used to going to aerobics or keep–fit classes, tell your instructor that you are pregnant She will advise you on when to ease up!
☆ Don't over-exhaust yourself.
☆ If you feel strained or experience pain, stop for a few moments or switch to something more gentle.
☆ If you haven't exercised much before, build up gradually — sudden strenuous exercise isn't good for anyone.

EXERCISE IN PREGNANCY

Ante-natal exercise classes are an excellent idea. These classes, which are usually run in the hospital, local clinic or by the National Childbirth Trust (see page 89) will help you learn movements which will enable you to avoid aches and pains as you get bigger. They will also help with some of the physical discomforts of pregnancy, such as indigestion, constipation, piles, incontinence and difficulty in sleeping. Ask about the classes at the hospital or ask your midwife, GP or health visitor where your nearest ones are held. If you cannot get to a class there are several helpful books which show how to do pregnancy exercises at home (see page 91).

A few women are advised not to exercise during pregnancy. This may be because they have a past history of miscarriages or other pregnancy complications. If you are concerned about the safety of any exercise, check with your doctor.

LOOK AFTER YOUR BACK!

There is a great temptation to adopt a slouching posture when you become pregnant. If you allow yourself to sag, then the latter stages of pregnancy will be more uncomfortable because of the extra strain on your back.

Try to remember to:

1. Stand tall and consciously straighten your spine.

2. Sit with your back supported.

3. When you carry things hold them close to your body.

4. When getting up from the floor, bend your knees and turn to the side and push up.

5. Start to do household chores such as ironing, and preparing vegetables, sitting down.

LOOK AFTER YOUR BACK!

6. Sit beside the washbasin and use a shampoo hose when washing your hair.

7. Lie still for a while and listen to your breathing.

8. When you get up, do it slowly and calmly, easing your way back into the activities of the rest of the day.

Pregnancy is a time for pampering yourself. After all, once the baby has arrived there won't be much time to do so! So here are some things that you can enjoy during the months of waiting:

☆ Enjoy a long soak in a warm (not too hot) bath.
☆ Ask your partner to massage you using oil or baby lotion. This is also good during labour, so start practising.
☆ Go to the hairdresser and have a new style — it is not a good time for a perm though.
☆ Go to museums, art galleries and other places that you have been meaning to go to for ages.
☆ Buy some jewellery to brighten up one of your maternity dresses.
☆ Go to a big store and volunteer for a make-up.

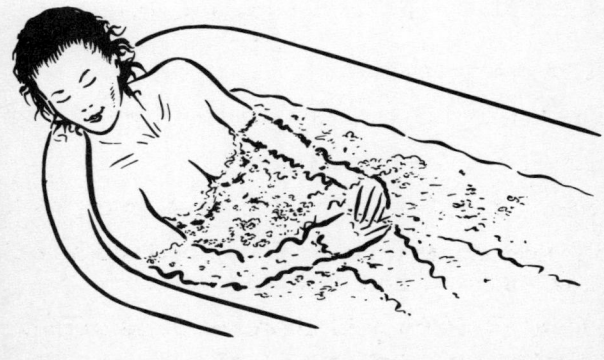

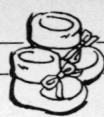

PREGNANCY WORRIES

It may well be the first time that you have been pregnant, so you may not know what is normal and what is not. What may be a small concern to a doctor or midwife may be a big problem to you. Whatever it is, help starts here, with advice on prevention as well as home remedies for minor problems.

PREVENTION OF PROBLEMS

Knowing what problems can occur can make you more keen to prevent them. Haemorrhoids (piles) for instance, can be made a lot worse by constipation. Constipation also makes you feel bloated and uncomfortable, so what can be done to prevent it happening in the first place? Diet plays an important part, so eat plenty of fresh fruit and vegetables. Fibre, such as that found in many breakfast cereals, or added to food — for instance, bran, will also help. Drink plenty of water and fruit juice. If you have to resort to laxatives use a natural product such as Senokot, but only if all else fails.

Backache is another thing that can be prevented by exercise and correcting your posture when you are standing (see ch. 3).

For most of the minor problems of pregnancy there are things that you can do to help yourself. If, however, the problem persists, mention it to your midwife or doctor.

RELAXATION

Relaxation is important at all times of our lives, but the technique is often not learnt until you go to ante-natal classes. Once you have a baby it will be more difficult for you to lie and soak in the bath for half an hour, so you have to learn other ways to ease stress and tension.

One of the most difficult things is to completely relax your mind and your body. If you use the 'relaxation' time to plan your shopping or the weekend's meals then you are **not** relaxing. Many people find it easier to relax whilst listening to soothing music, others prefer total silence.

Here is my recipe for relaxing:

1. Take enough pillows or cushions to make you comfortable.
2. Find the best position for you, back, side or propped up.
3. Shut your eyes and take some slow deep breaths.
4. Think about your body starting at your feet. Tense your feet then relax them, then move on to your knees, calves, thighs and so on until you finish with your face.
5. Keep breathing slowly and deeply and feel the tension draining out of you.

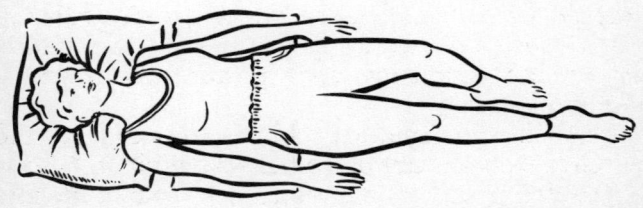

PREGNANCY PROBLEMS

Why caused?	*Help*
BACKACHE	
Bad posture or, later on, it may be due to the baby pressing on the spinal area. In some cases this causes sciatica which needs treatment by an obstetric physiotherapist. Progesterone, a hormone which is active during pregnancy, causes softening of the ligaments and joints of the lower back in readiness for labour.	Exercise of the right sort will help strengthen and support your back (see p. 28). Swimming is also relaxing and helpful. Make sure the mattress on your bed is firm — if not put a board under your side. Wear low or flat shoes. When travelling, walk around for a few minutes each hour.
BLADDER PROBLEMS	
The uterus presses on the bladder as it enlarges in early pregnancy. Later, the baby's head, when in the pelvis, also causes pressure on the bladder.	Tea, coffee and alcohol, especially beer, make you want to urinate more often so avoid these especially at night. Remember to go the lavatory before you go out and before doing any strenuous exercise.

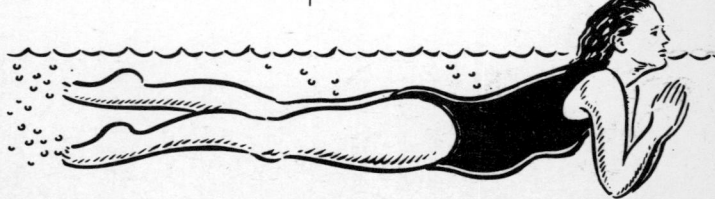

PREGNANCY PROBLEMS

Why caused?	*Help*
Cystitis: This is an infection of the bladder and urethra (the tube from the bladder to outside). It is often experienced during pregnancy because the higher levels of the hormone progesterone relax the bladder muscles allowing it to become infected more easily. Cystitis gives a burning sensation when you urinate and makes you feel as if you want to go all the time.	If you have suffered from cystitis in the past, make sure that you drink plenty during pregnancy. At least 600 ml/1 pint every hour in the early stages of pregnancy may prevent it becoming worse. Bad cystitis needs treatment from your GP. It can lead to a high temperature and a great deal of pain. Your urine will be checked at the antenatal clinic for signs of infection.
Incontinence: Again caused by the hormone progesterone relaxing the muscles of the bladder and urethra. The Braxton Hicks contractions can also cause slight incontinence in later pregnancy.	Make sure that you do not have an infection and, if you suspect that you may have one, get it treated. It may help if you wear a pantie liner — this will protect you if you have 'dribble' problems when you sneeze! Practise your pelvic floor exercises and avoid becoming constipated.

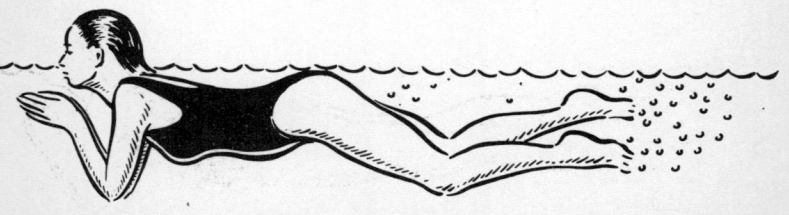

PREGNANCY PROBLEMS

Why caused?	*Help*
DISCHARGE	
Vaginal discharge is common in pregnancy. It is normally clear or white and does not smell offensive. *Thrush* is caused by a change in the acidity of the vagina. It will cause a thick white or yellow discharge and extreme itchiness which stings when you urinate. Thrush is also caused by stress and being run down, and is common in diabetics.	Wear cotton pants and, if necessary, a pantie liner. Thrush can be easily treated by pessaries or cream from the doctor. Your partner should also use the cream if the problem recurs after treatment. Thrush can be prevented by wearing cotton underwear and avoiding tight clothes. Do not soak in hot baths and wash with unscented products.
Trichomonas: will also cause a discharge and infection. It is acquired from your partner during sexual intercourse.	Treatment, in the form of pessaries or cream and antibiotics for both of you, will clear it up. While treatment is under way use a condom to prevent re-infection.
FAINTING	
A feeling of dizziness, or fainting, can happen in early pregnancy and is a circulation problem. The womb and baby need a large supply of blood and sometimes, particularly after exercise, the brain is momentarily a bit short of blood and you feel faint. Standing still makes the problem worse.	Try not to stand still for long periods and take care when you stand up after sitting. Ask for a seat on the bus or train. Occasionally you may feel faint when lying on your back; if so, turn on to your side. This is caused by the baby lying on your main blood vessels in the low back area.

PREGNANCY PROBLEMS

Why caused?	*Help*
HEADACHES	
Headaches are caused by bad posture, tension or heavy colds. Pregnant women are advised not to take unnecessary medication during pregnancy as this may pass to the baby. If headaches persist, tell your GP or midwife.	Fresh air, exercise and relaxation will all help. Take a look at yourself in a mirror or shop window and check your posture. If a headache is a problem, and it is vital for you to be on top form, two paracetamol are considered fairly safe. Severe headaches can be a sign of high blood pressure.
INDIGESTION	
Indigestion is caused by your enlarged womb pressing on your stomach and intestines. It is also thought to be affected by high levels of the hormone progesterone relaxing the valve at the top of the stomach. Certain foods can make it feel worse.	Indigestion is relieved by eating smaller meals more often and sitting up well. Do not eat too late at night and try to avoid foods that seem to make it worse. Avoid indigestion tablets. Milk of Magnesia can be helpful. Heartburn can be relieved by a drink of milk or herbal tea. If it happens at night try to sleep propped up. Sometimes iron tablets can be the cause. Speak to your doctor about this.

PREGNANCY PROBLEMS

| *Why caused?* | *Help* |

NAUSEA, SICKNESS

Again, hormone changes are the cause of these problems, though many women are not affected. Others experience nausea with one pregnancy and not with the next. It really can make you ask 'Is it all worth it?' but for most women it will go by about 14 weeks of pregnancy. Some feel sick all day, some in the morning and some in the evenings.

It is difficult to cure nausea, but it is worth trying some of the following which have helped others:
* Eat small meals frequently
* Keep a snack handy
* Avoid food and smells that make you fell worse
* Have a milky drink at night and have a snack by your bedside in case you wake up
* Try high carbohydrate diet, i.e. rice, bread, potatoes
* Iron tablets may be a problem. Ask for enteric coated ones.

Morning sickness: nibble a dry biscuit before you even lift your head from the pillow, get up slowly and have a peppermint tea or suck some candied ginger.

Evening sickness: try not to get overtired — have a rest after lunch if you can and rest again when you get in from work. Avoid cooking if at all possible.

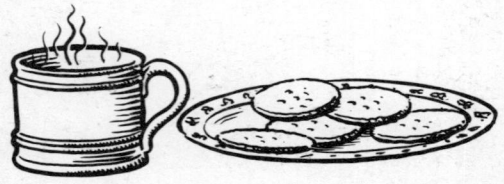

PREGNANCY PROBLEMS

Why caused?	*Help*
PILES AND VARICOSE VEINS	

Piles are varicose veins around the rectum and anus. The veins may become congested because the heart is having to work extra hard to supply the uterus. Piles may become worse as the baby gets bigger and they may bleed or stick out.

Constipation makes piles a lot worse as does straining when you go to the lavatory.

Varicose veins are also caused by the pressure of the baby's head on the blood vessels in your legs. Both piles and varicose veins usually disappear after pregnancy.

Eat plenty of fresh fruit and vegetables, and drink plenty. Some people find sitting on an ice pack (or small pack of frozen peas kept for the purpose) soothing.

If the piles stick out, push them back in using a little vaseline. Sometimes an anaesthetic cream may help the itching. Varicose veins are made worse by standing or sitting with your legs crossed. Try to rest with your feet raised and exercise your legs and feet as much as possible. Support tights are good but they must be put on *before* you stand up.

Vulval varicose veins are most uncomfortable. Try sleeping with a pillow under your bottom. Some find a pad held on with an old-fashioned sanitary belt helps to ease the swollen feeling.

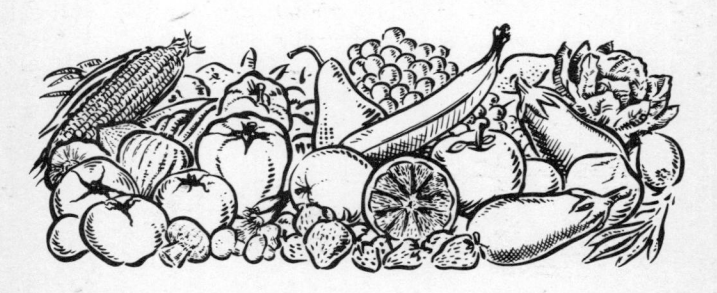

PREGNANCY PROBLEMS

Why caused?	*Help*
SLEEPLESSNESS	
In early pregnancy this may be caused by you needing to empty your bladder frequently or later because the baby is kicking a lot. You may feel uncomfortably hot and sweaty. Bad dreams are common in the later states of pregnancy.	Make sure you take some exercise every day. Before bed, have a warm bath and practise your relaxation exercises. If you feel uncomfortable, try using a pillow to support your back. If you feel worried about labour, talk to a midwife, friend or your partner. Some women find hawthorn flowers, which can be bought and made into a herbal tea, helpful.
SWELLING	
Swelling in pregnancy is often seen in the ankles, hands and feet particularly at the end of the day, when the weather is hot or if you have been sitting for a long time. Fluid gathers in the lower parts of the body and is not pumped away as quickly as usual.	Try to rest with your legs raised every afternoon and avoid standing or sitting for long periods without a walk. Comfortable shoes will help. Some women find a half size larger is useful for wearing at home in the evening. Always mention any swelling to your midwife or doctor, as it can also be a sign of pre-eclampsia (see page 90).

PREGNANCY PROBLEMS

Why caused?	*Help*
TIREDNESS	
Tiredness in early pregnancy is depressing — few people know that you are pregnant; there is nothing different about your appearance and you feel exhausted. Usually it passes off at about 12 weeks, but it will make life difficult, especially if you experience nausea or have other children to care for.	Get your partner or friends to help you, especially with shopping. Ask for someone to pack for you in the supermarket. Decide which things really need doing and forget the rest — they are not important and can wait. Try to talk to others about how you are feeling.

Many women who do not want to take drugs during pregnancy turn to homoeopathic remedies; for further information contact the British Homoeopathic Association (see page 88). Alternative medical practitioners, such as acupuncturists, chiropractors and so on are rarely mentioned by conventional medical practitioners. Before going for a consultation, talk to other mothers who have used them. Some GPs offer alternative therapies.

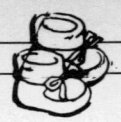

YOUR DEVELOPING BABY

Once you know that you are pregnant, your thoughts will naturally turn to your baby. You will wonder what the baby within you is actually like. Is it perfectly formed from the moment of conception, or do various parts form at different stages of the pregnancy? This week-by-week guide will give you an idea of what is happening inside your womb, and will help you to understand why certain tests are done at specific times.

Seven days after fertilization the egg (ovum) embeds itself in the body of the uterus. It starts to divide, but is not yet a foetus.

Week 4: The embryo is just visible to the naked eye and menstruation ceases because of the rising levels of the hormone progesterone. The progesterone also thickens the lining of the uterus into which the outer layer of cells sends root-like branches which will form the placenta.

Week 5: The foetus is beginning to take shape and a definite head and 'tail' develop. The nervous system has started to be formed together with the spine and brain.

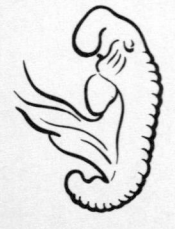

Week 5

Week 6: The head and chest are forming together with the abdominal cavity. The heart is forming and early circulation of blood is starting. The placenta begins to grow and the umbilical cord which contains the blood vessels which run between your circulatory system and the baby's are functioning. Already the tail is beginning to disappear and limb buds form at the four corners of the body. The baby has a neck, and the mouth and jaw are beginning to develop. The foetus is not 5 mm/¼ in long.

Week 7: The baby's head is beginning to form its own shape. It is rather lumpy with depressions where the ears and eyes are growing. The eyes appear as lumps covered in skin and nostrils appear, even though the nose is not yet formed. The arms and legs are more obvious now. By the end of this week the brain and spinal cord will be nearly complete. The liver, kidneys, lungs and intestines are formed but not functioning. The foetus is now 1 cm/½ in long.

Week 8: The heart is now pumping regularly and blood vessels can be seen through the transparent paper-like skin. The bones of the arms and legs are getting longer and harder, the toes and fingers are visible. The head of the foetus is large in comparison to the rest of the body, but the face is becoming recognizable. The mouth will start to open once the jaws are joined at the sides. The foetus is now 2.3 cm/⅞ in long.

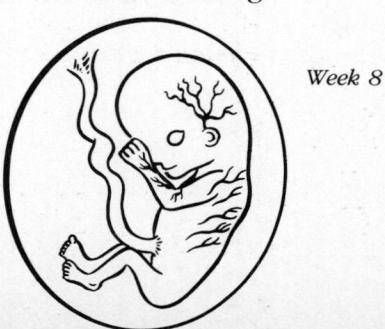

Week 8

YOUR DEVELOPING BABY

Week 9: The baby's head is still bent forward onto its chest and the eyes are now fully developed though shut. The nose has appeared and the inner ear is developing. Hands and feet are more obvious and movements can be seen though not felt by the mother. The foetus is now 2·5 cm/1 in long.

Week 10: The eyes have grown larger and the external part of the ear is starting to develop as the inner part is now completely formed. The umbilical cord is properly formed and blood is circulating. The internal organs continue to develop and the foetus is now 4.5 cm/1¾ in long.

Week 11: The foetus now looks like a small baby although its head is still large and its limbs are rather small. Limb and spine movements increase. The ovaries and testicles have formed, but the sex cannot yet be detected. The majority of the organs of the foetus are now formed and funtioning.

It is during these eleven weeks that most congenital abnormalities occur. Once the major organs have been formed the baby is unlikely to come to much harm. This is why it is so important to take great care of what you eat, drink and smoke in the early weeks of pregnancy. Eleven weeks is a short time to go without those substances which can cause so much harm to your developing baby.

Week 12: By this week you should be able to feel your uterus as a hard lump just above the pubic bone. The baby will now measure about 6.5 cm/2¾ in and weigh about 20 g/¾ oz. The face is now properly formed although the outer part of the ear is developing. The internal organs continue to grow and develop as the umbilical cord starts to circulate blood between the baby and the placenta.

YOUR DEVELOPING BABY

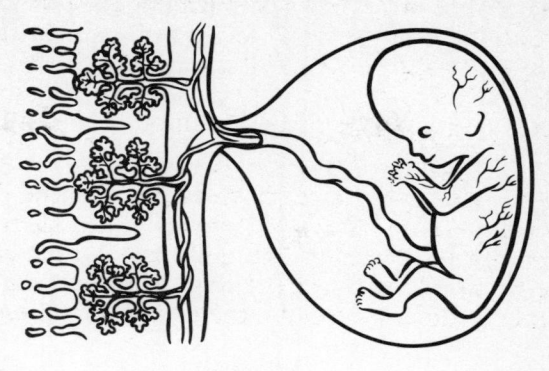

Week 13

Week 13: The baby is now properly formed, but if born would not be able to survive because its internal organs are insufficiently mature. The remainder of the pregnancy is necessary to allow the baby time to grow big enough to survive out of the womb. The baby is now 7.5 cm/ 3 in long and weighs 25 g/1 oz.

By Week 16: The baby will be making many active movements but, as yet, these are not felt by the mother. The sex of the baby can now be seen on ultrasound examination. The baby will be covered in fine hair and the eyebrows and eyelashes will start to grow. Your placenta will now be functioning well allowing the heart to beat strongly. The baby will drink some of the amniotic fluid which surrounds him and will pass a little urine as his kidneys start to work.

YOUR DEVELOPING BABY

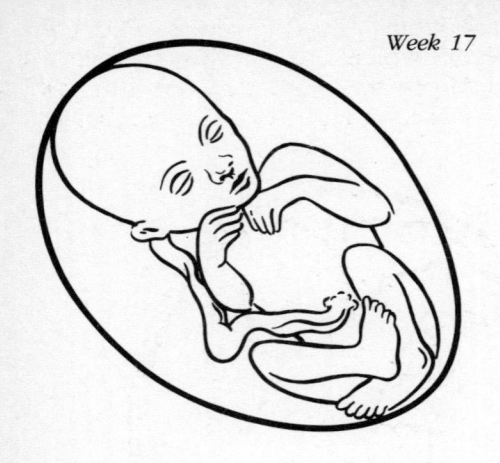

Week 17

By Week 18: About now you will start to feel your baby move. It may occur earlier if this is not your first pregnancy. Remember to note it so that you can tell the doctor or midwife. The baby is surrounded by amniotic fluid which protects him and allows him to move freely.

By Week 24: If the baby were born now it is possible that he would survive. He would need to spend a few months in the special care baby unit until his lungs were working well and he had grown to about 2.25 kg/5 lb. At 24 weeks the baby is about 32.5 cm/13 in long and weighs about 500 g/18 oz.

Week 28: The baby is now considered by paediatricians to be 'viable' or capable of a life outside the womb. A baby born at this time must be registered. His lungs are working quite well although he may have some breathing problems outside the womb.

The midwife will be able to feel the baby's position in your womb and determine if he or she is head down or

YOUR DEVELOPING BABY

in the breech (bottom down) position. The baby is covered with vernix which is a greasy substance which protects the skin from the amniotic fluid. The baby is about 37 cm/14½ in long and weighs about 900 g/2 lb.

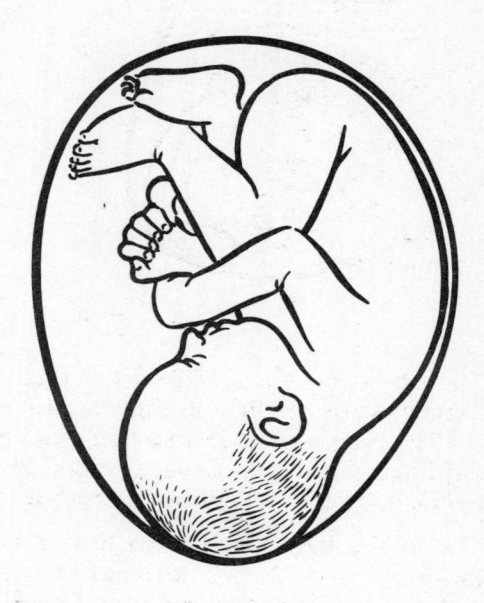

Week 28

By 36 Weeks: The baby is perfectly formed and the size of the head is now in proportion to the rest of the body. A baby delivered at 36 weeks stands more than a 90 per cent chance of survival. The baby will be in its final birth position with the head or bottom going down into the pelvis. The baby will weigh about 2.5 kg/5½ lb and be roughly 45 cm/18 in long.

YOUR DEVELOPING BABY

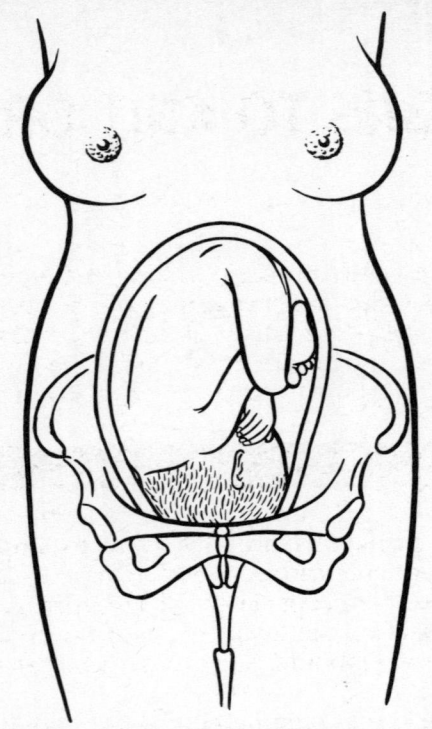

Your baby's head has dropped into your pelvis

Week 40: This is the normal length of a full-term pregnancy. The baby will be well developed and have enough fat to round the arms and legs. The hairy covering will have almost disappeared, but the vernix or fat will still be seen especially in the skin creases.

Babies are always born with blue eyes but, over the first few months, the colour will change. At 40 weeks the average baby will be 50 cm/20 in long and weigh 3.4 kg/ 7 lb 6 oz.

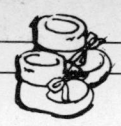

DESIGNS TO KNIT OR SEW

Many of the lovely nursery designs and equipment that you see in shops and magazines can be copied if you have time and some artistic ability. The following ideas for baby and you are easy to make and will be rewarding for you to use once your baby has arrived.

1. PATCHWORK BLANKET

Even if you are not a brilliant knitter a knitted patchwork blanket is an ideal way to improve your skills! The squares can be any size you decide, but are most effective if kept fairly small, that is less than 10 cm/4 in. You can use scraps of wool donated by friends and neighbours, so it need not cost much.

Use size 4½ mm knitting needles and double-knitting wool. The tension should be 10 stitches to 5 cm/2 in. Cast on required number of stitches (25 stitches for 13 cm/5 in square) and knit 50 rows or until your piece is square. Cast off loosely. Make more squares in the same way. Most cot blankets are usually 120 cm/48 in square, but you can make yours to fit your cot, crib or pram exactly. Join the squares together using one colour wool and an embroidery needle or bodkin.

Finishing: You can either leave the knitting as it is, or bind the edges to give it a more attractive finish. Choose either satin ribbon or a matching braid (available from

2. BABY EQUIPMENT HOLDER

most drapery departments). For a firmer more durable blanket you could also think of lining it before you bind the edges. Old flannelette sheeting can be used for lining.

2. BABY EQUIPMENT HOLDER

You will be amazed at the number of lotions, creams, powders and so on that you acquire when you have a baby. It is more convenient to keep them all together in a holder, so that they are handy when you need them. (Make sure that you do not use the holder for medicines.) One of the most useful types of holder is a plastic tool tidy that can be bought from department stores. This can be brightened up by stencilling. It is good because, if anything leaks or spills, it an easily be scrubbed out.

Small baskets are also a good idea, but not quite so practical, but lined with quilted material they look very pretty.

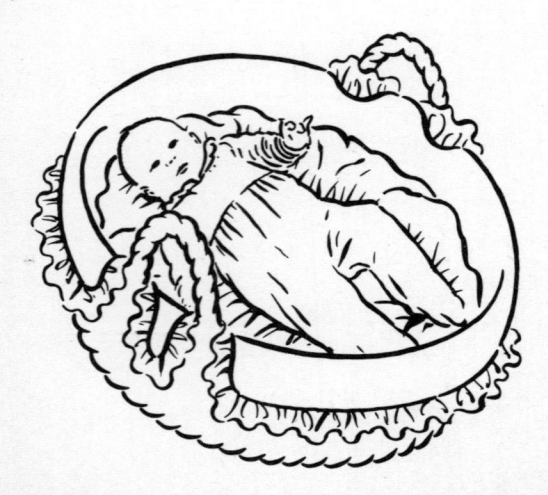

2. BABY EQUIPMENT HOLDER

To cover the bottom of the basket measure the width and length of the inside of the basket. Add 2.5 cm/1 in to each measure to allow for turnings and from your fabric cut a rectangle or circle to these measurements. Place the fabric inside the basket, right side up, and press into the edges of the base, where it joins the sides, and mark the exact outline of the base with pins. Trim the fabric to 1 cm/½ in from the pin line. Fold the fabric in two, right sides facing, and mark the centre line on the wrong side of the fabric.

To line the sides of the basket, measure the inside depth of the basket and double it. Cut two pieces of fabric each the basket depth measurement and half the length of the basket. With right sides together join the two pieces at the short ends, forming a circle, with 1 cm/½ in seams. Press open. Turn up the seam allowance along the bottom edge and notch into it all the way round. Then join the side section to the bottom section, right sides facing. (See figure 1.)

Next, put the lining in position in the basket and, using pins, mark the position of any handles and the rim of the basket. Remove the lining from the basket and fold in

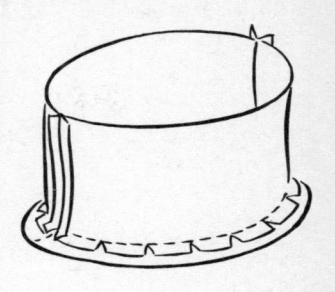

Figure 1

half lengthwise. On each side draw a line down from each of the pins marking the handle, placing the lines at right angles to the pin line, marking the top edge of the basket, and taking the line to the edge of the fabric. Join the lines with curves and round off the lower edge of the outer lines. (See figure 2.)

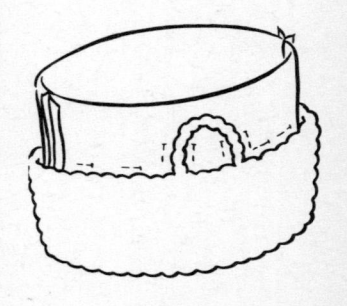

Figure 2

2. BABY EQUIPMENT HOLDER

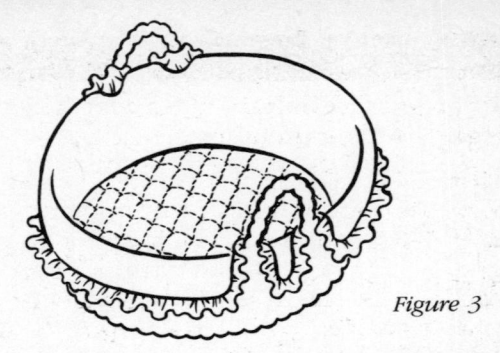

Figure 3

Finally, cut the lining as marked and bind the raw edge. Put the lining in the basket folding the surplus over the edge and slotting it through the handles.

A more decorative finish may be achieved by making a double ruffle. Cut the length of fabric required (between one and a half and twice the finished length required) with twice the desired finished width. Fold the strip in half lengthwise and make two lines of tacking through the double thickness. The top edge can be finished off with a zigzag stitch through all thicknesses or with a self-bound edge.

This process can also be used to line a Moses Basket. These baskets are useful for around the house for the baby to sleep in. Remember, though, not to leave the basket on a floor where there is underfloor central heating and never leave it on a table where it may be knocked off. These baskets are also not safe in cars as they cannot be secured properly.

3. CHANGING BAG

A large padded bag with shoulder–length handles which unzips to provide a useful changing mat.

You will need 70 cm/28 in × 90 cm/36 in coloured fabric;
50 cm/20 in × 90 cm/36 in plastic sheeting;
70 cm/28 in × 90 cm/36 in medium weight wadding;
5 m/5.4 yd of 17 mm/¾ in wide bias binding;
two zips 40 cm/16 in long and thread to match

Cut from both the fabric and the wadding one piece 45 × 80 cm/18 × 32 in and two pieces 90 × 10 cm/36 × 4 in.

From plastic sheeting cut one piece 45 × 80 cm/18 × 32 in.

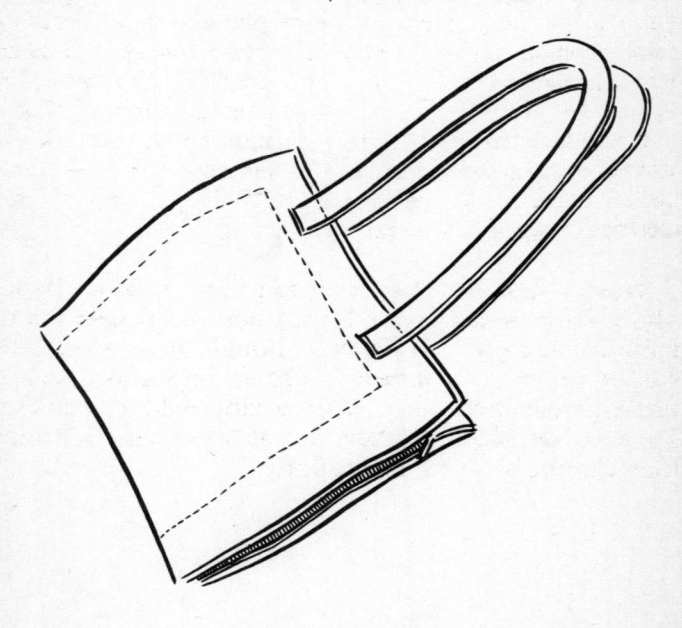

3. CHANGING BAG

Layer and stitch fabric, wadding and plastic sheeting and then apply bias binding around all edges. Stitch a line of quilting around the bag 7.5 cm/3 in from all edges.

Alternatively stitch other quilting patterns as desired. Sew zips in position down each side of bag. Working with zip open and teeth level with edge of bias binding fold tapes under at open end to neaten and stitch zip in place.

Work from top to bottom on each side turning any spare length inwards at fold of bag. Sew in place finishing about 2 cm/¾ in from bottom of bag. Stitch bottom of zip in place leaving sufficient loose zip to allow bag to open out flat. Pin or tack the wadding to both handle pieces. Trim 2 cm/¾ in from the ends of each piece of wadding and turn material up to enclose wadding, pinning or tacking in place. Fold each handle in half lengthways and, with raw edges even, sew together though all layers as close to edge as possible. Trim close to stitching. Apply bias binding. Pin or tack handles in place on each side of bag, lapping 7.5 cm/3 in of handle over bag and positioning each handle 11 cm/4½ in from outside edge. Stitch in place sewing close to edge of handles through all layers.

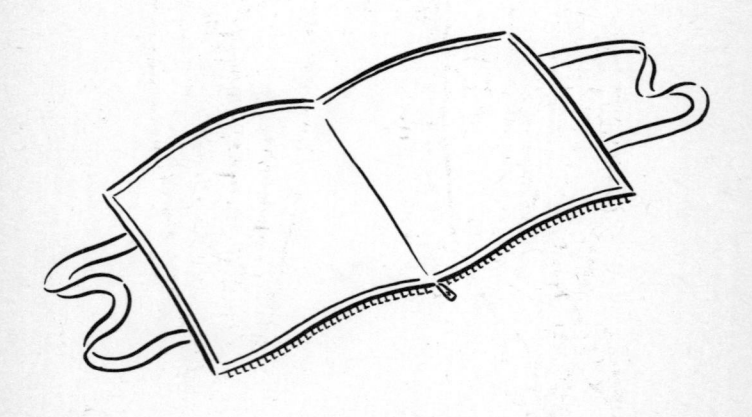

EASY DUNGAREE PATTERN

HERE IS AN EASY DUNGAREE PATTERN FOR YOU TO MAKE

This easy and comfortable outfit is great for everyday wear, providing that you are in reasonably good shape. They can, however, if you are not careful, make you look rather big and be a bit unflattering. Never wear

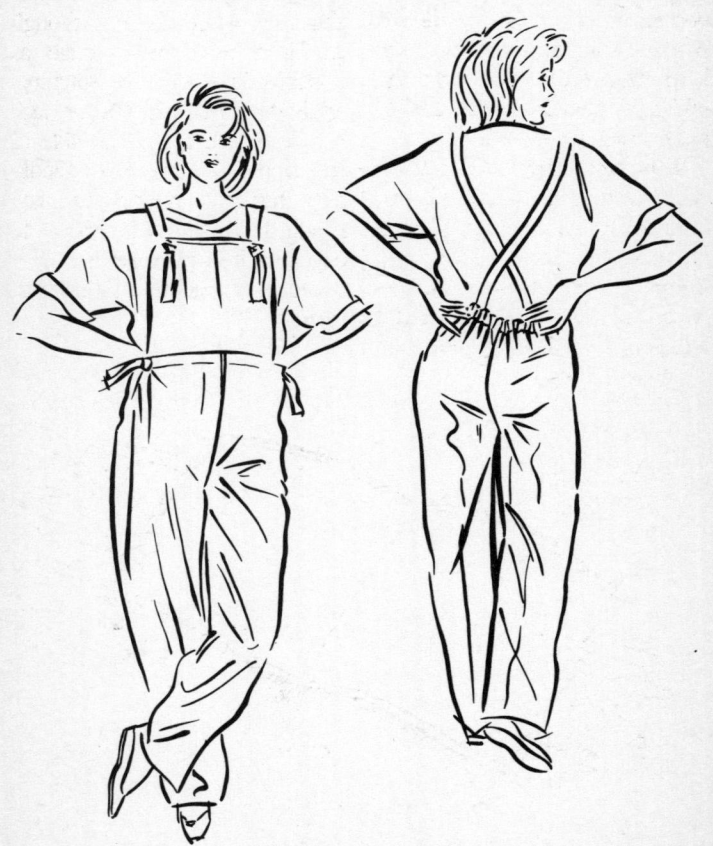

EASY DUNGAREE PATTERN

them when they are so tight that they are pulling over the tummy. They are ideal for summer made in heavy cotton, such as a cotton drill or cotton ticking. For winter, choose needlecord or denim, but do make sure that the fabric you choose it not so stiff as to make the dungarees uncomfortable — with heavier fabrics, it sometimes pays to wash them before sewing. Dungarees go well with shirts, sweaters or T-shirts, but don't overload yourself.

Size:
to fit size 8–10, 12–14, 16–18 (normal sizes).

Materials:
2.60 m/2⅞ yd of 90 cm/36 in wide fabric.
40 cm/16 in of 2 cm/¾ in wide elastic.
Matching thread.

Cutting out:
following the graph pattern to make a paper pattern using dressmakers' 5 cm/2 in squared pattern paper. Follow cutting layout for sizes 8–10 and 12–14. For size 16–18, cut out bib first on folded fabric. Cut remaining fabric in half widthwise so you have two pieces 115 cm × 90 cm/46 in × 36 in and lay one half on top of the other, right sides facing. Lay back pattern piece to one side (left), reverse front and lay next to back (right). Fit in straps and ties alongside.

Seam allowances of 15 mm/⅝ in are included in the pattern.

Making up
Make 22 mm/⅞ in vertical buttonholes in fronts where marked with top of buttonhole exactly 37 mm/ 1⅜ in below upper raw edge. (If liked reinforce wrong side with a square of Iron-On Vilene beforehand.)

Pin and stitch one front to one back at side and inside leg seams, right sides facing: press open. Repeat with other leg. Turn leg to right side and slot inside other leg, matching centre fronts, centre backs and inside leg seams. Pin and stitch crotch seam, right sides facing, stitch again 6 mm/¼ in inside first stitching and trim seam allowances close to second stitching. Overcase edges together and press seam to one side except under crutch.

Pin and stitch both bib pieces

EASY DUNGAREE PATTERN

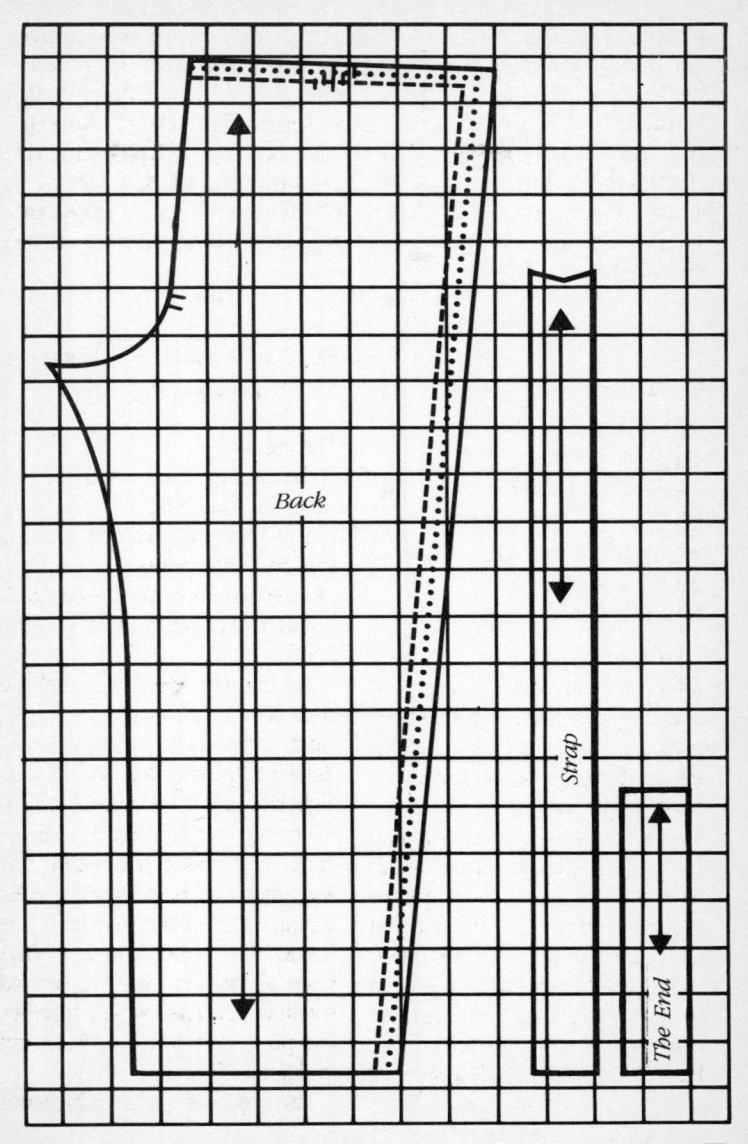

Back

Strap

The End

EASY DUNGAREE PATTERN

- - - - - Size 8 – 10
· · · · · Size 12 – 14
——— Size 16 – 18
⟵⟶ Grain of Fabric

Buttonhole Position

Front

Buttonholes

Bib

Centre Front

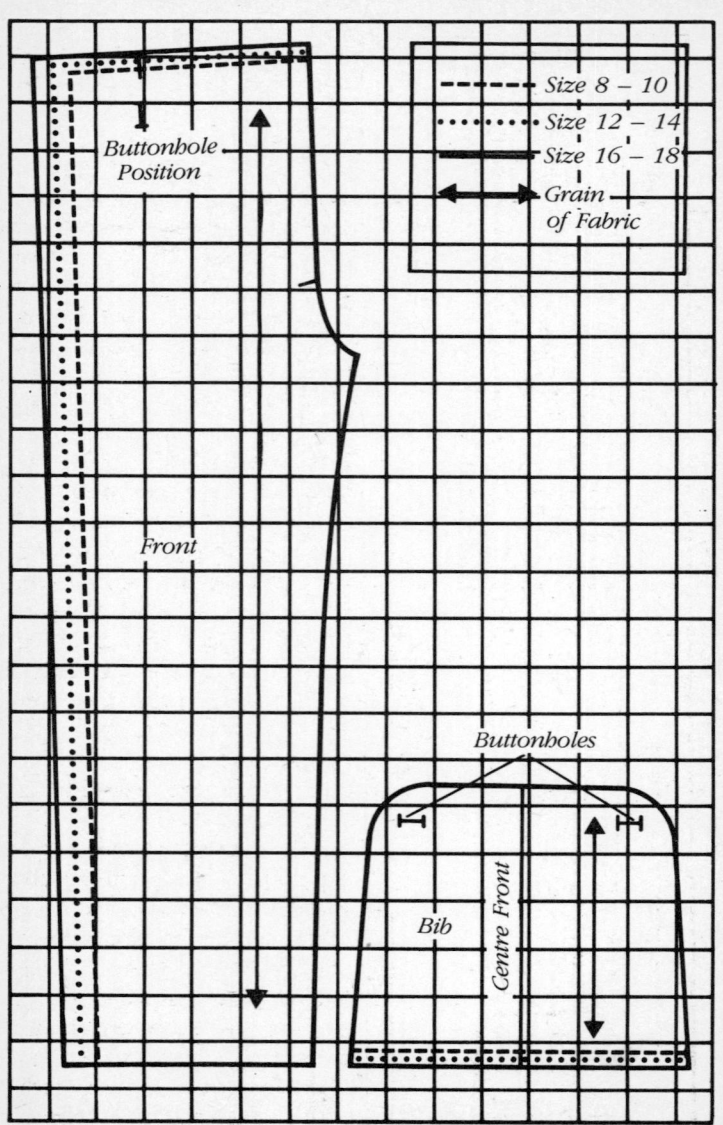

1 grid square = 5 cm (2 in)

EASY DUNGAREE PATTERN

Cutting Layout

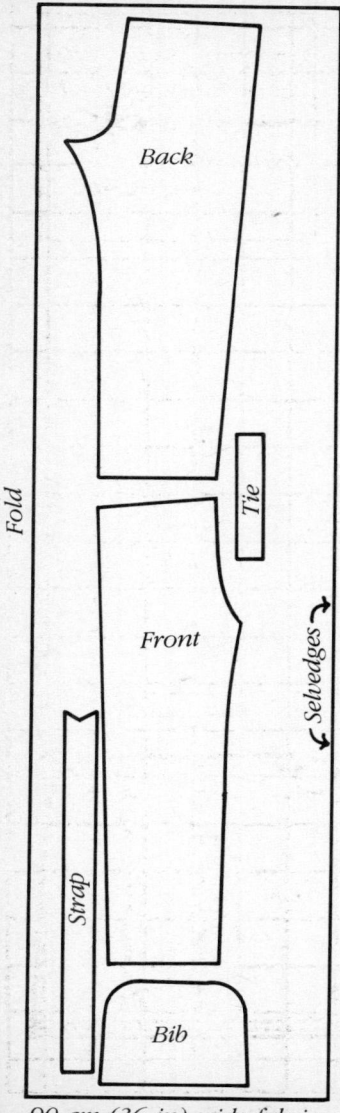

Fold

Back

Tie

Front

Selvedges

Strap

Bib

90 cm (36 in) wide fabric

together, right side facing, leaving lower edge open. Trim seam allowances, clip curves, and turn to right side: press. Top-stitch close to finished edges and again 1 cm/3/8 in from edge: tack lower edges together. Make two horizontal buttonholes 22 mm/7/8 in long where marked. Pin bib to front of pants in between front buttonholes, right sides facing, and tack in place 6 m/1/4 in from edge. Stitch in place 35 mm/1¼ in from edge.

Make straps by folding in half lengthwise, right sides inside, and stitching along straight end and long edge. Trim seam allowances and corners and turn to right side: press and top-stitch close to all finished edges. Pin unfinished slanted ends to right side of back of pants where marked, so they 'lean' towards centre back, and tack in place 6 mm/1/4 in from edge. Stitch in place 35 mm/1¼ in from edge.

Press under remaining top edge of pants by 35 mm/1¼ in and top-stitch 25 mm/1 in from fold.

Make tie ends by folding ties in half lengthwise, right sides inside, and stitching along one short and the long edge. Trim seam allowances and corners and turn to right side: press and top-stitch close to all finished edges. Overlap

KNITS FOR BABY

unfinished ends and elastic ends by 1 cm/⅜ in and stitch securely. Slot tie through buttonholes into upper casing so that ties extend through buttonholes.

Turn up 15 mm/⅝ in hem and press: top-stitch in place 1 cm/⅜ in from fold.

Slot strap ends through buttonholes in bib and knot.

KNITS FOR BABY

This little outfit is easy to knit in garter stitch. Follow the washing instructions supplied on the wool band.

Materials
5, 50 g (1¾ oz) balls of Emu Superwash DK or other DK in Cream (A), 1 ball each of Blue (B), Green (C), Grey (D) and Yellow (E).
3 buttons and elastic for trousers.
1 pair each of 3¼ mm (No 10) and 4 mm (No 8) needles.
1 crochet hook

Measurements
To fit approx 6–12 months.
chest 50 cm/20 in. Sleeve seam 21.5 cm/8½ in. Inside leg 22.5 cm/9½ in.

Tension
20 sts and 40 rows to 10 cm (4 in) over g. st using 4 mm (No 8) needles.

Abbreviations
K-knit; p-purl; st(s)-stitches; g. st-garter stitch; inc-increase; dec-decrease; beg-beginning; sl-slip; WS-wrong side; RS-right side; rep-repeat; patt-pattern; cont-continue.

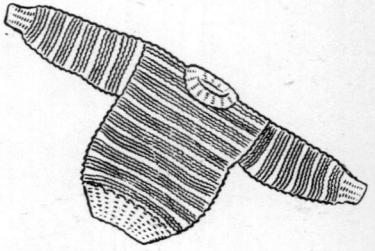

SWEATER

Front
*With 3¼ mm (No 10) needles and A cast on 46 sts.
1st row: K3 (p2, k2) to last st, k1.
2nd row: K1, (p2, k2) to last 3 sts, p2, k1.
Cont working in rib for 12 more rows.
Change to 4 mm (No 8) needles and work in stripe patt as follows:
2 rows in B, 2 rows in C, 2 rows in D, 2 rows in E then 2 rows in A.

KNITS FOR BABY

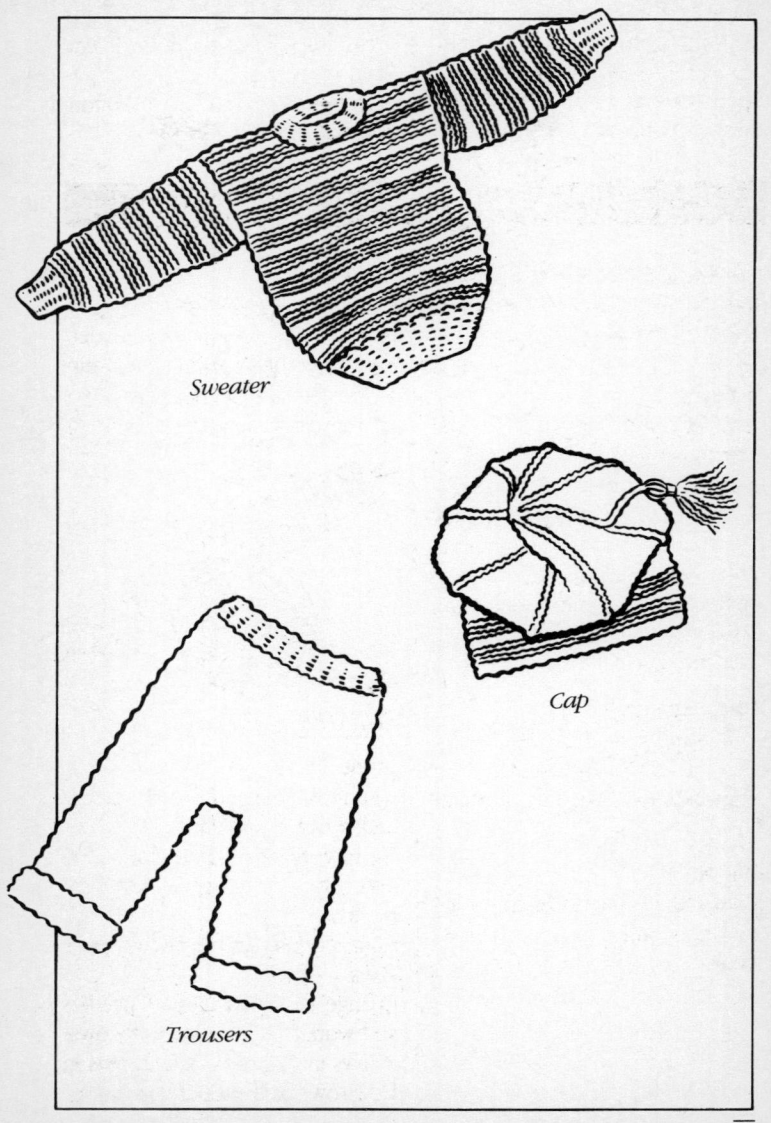

Sweater

Cap

Trousers

KNITS FOR BABY

Cont working this patt until work measures 24.5 cm/10 in.

Neck Shaping
Next row: K 19, turn (cont on these sts).
Dec 1 st on neck at next 4 rows.
Then work 11 rows. Casting off, slip centre 8 sts on a spare needle.
Next row: K.
Then complete as first half.

Back
Work as for Front until Back measures same as Front to shoulder.
Next row: Cast off 30 sts loosely, k to end.
Next row: Cast off 4 sts loosely, k to end.

Work 6 rows on remaining stitches for underwrap and then cast off.

Sleeves
With 3¼ mm (No 10) needles and A cast on 28 sts.
Work in rib for 12 rows inc by 4 sts evenly on last row.
Change to 4 mm (No 8) needles and working in g. st, and stripe patt as set, work 10 rows. Inc 1 st at each end of next row and then on every following 8th row until you have 40 sts.
Cont knitting until sleeve measures 19 cm/7½ in. Work 12 rows in patt and then cast off.

Neckband
Sew right shoulder seam. On outside of work join 7 sts on left shoulder. Using 3¼ mm (No 10) needles and A, k 10 sts, down left front neck, k across centre sts inc 2 sts evenly, k 10 sts up right front neck, k up 18 sts from back neck and 4 sts from underwrap.
Work 5 rows in rib and cast off loosely.

To make up
Sew in sleeves then join side seams. Work 3 buttonhole loops on front left shoulder, sew buttons to correspond.

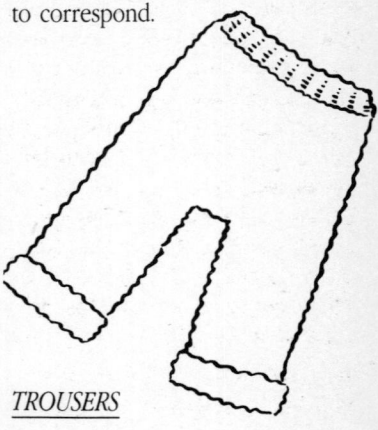

TROUSERS

Front
*With 4 mm (No 8) needles and A cast on 20 sts. Working in g. st, k for 20 cm/8 in then slip sts on a spare needle.
Work second leg to match.
Next row: K to end, cast on 8 sts

for crotch and k across sts on spare needle: 48 sts.

Cont working in g. st until work measures 16 cm (6½ in) measuring from the crotch and ending on a RS row. At the same time dec 2 sts on last row: 46 sts*.

with 3¼ mm (No 10) needles work 6 rows in rib, then cast off.

Back

Work as Front from * to * avoiding dec at the end of the last row.

1st row: K to last 3 sts, turn.
2nd row: Sl 1, k to last 3 sts, turn.
3rd and 4th rows: Sl 1, k to last 6 sts, turn.
5th and 6th rows: Sl 1, k to last 9 sts, turn.
7th and 8th rows: Sl 1, k to last 12 sts, turn.
9th and 10th rows: Sl 1, k to last 15 sts, turn.
11th row: Sl 1, k to last 16 sts, turn.
12th row: Sl 1, knit to end, dec 2 sts.

Then continue working as for Front from ** to **.

To make up

Join the side seams and sew in elastic at waist. Roll up trouser hems if desired.

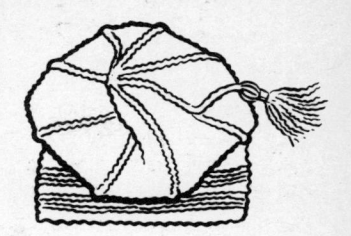

CAP

With 4 mm (No 8) needles and A cast on 81 sts. Work 20 rows in g. st using stripe patt as set for sweater.

Then cont in A only.

20th row: K.
21st row: K1, p to last st, k1.
Repeat these 2 rows 4 times then the 20th row once.

1st row: *k9, inc 1, rep from * to last st, k1.
2nd and alternate rows: K1, p to last st, K1.
3rd row: *K10, inc 1, rep from * to last st, k1.
5th row: *K11, inc 1, rep from * to last st, k1.
7th row: *K12, inc 1, rep from * to last st, k1.

Cont until there are 137 st.

Work 3 cm/1¼ in without shaping, ending with a p row.

1st row: K1, *k15, k2 tog, rep from * to end of row.
2nd and alternate rows: K1, p to last st, k1.
3rd row: K1, *k14, k2 tog, rep from * to end of row.

5th row: K1, *k13, k2 tog, rep from * to end of row.
7th row: K1, *k12, k2 tog, rep from * to end of row.
Cont until 17 sts remain, ending with a p row.
Next row: K1, *k2 tog, rep from * to end of row.

To make up
Sew up seam. Make a crochet chain and fasten to the top of the cap attaching the tassel to the end using strands from all the coloured yarns.

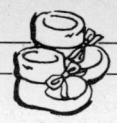

MAKING YOUR HOME READY

If you enjoy making things or have creative ideas, pregnancy is the time to make the most of it. Once you have given up work there are many things that you can start to think about and make.

Looking ahead you will need to make sure that your cupboards and freezer, if you have one, are well stocked. A new baby is a full–time occupation, so it is wonderful to feel that, at least for the first week or two, you have enough food in the house. Accept all offers of help from family or friends. Here are some ideas:

☆ Prepare a shopping list of perishable items, such as fruit, vegetables, bread and dairy produce, that your partner or friends can get in ready for your return home.

☆ Stock the freezer with ready meals.

☆ If a friend offers help, ask for a home-made cake or casserole.

☆ Perhaps a friend might be prepared to have the baby for a few hours while you catch up on sleep.

It may seem a bit calculating to start thinking in this way before the baby is even born, but, in reality, having a new baby is tiring and the more help you can get the better you will be able to cope. Many women, looking back over the first year after the birth of their baby, admit that they felt depressed, tired and confused in the first few months and that they did not ask for enough help. Society today expects women to cope with life without the support that was available years ago. Women go back to work, or are working part time, in order to meet the family's financial needs. The image to which we aspire is portrayed in magazines and on television as the Jack–of–all–trades SuperMum which is hard, if not impossible to achieve without a great deal of help. So, throw out all your ideas of life being the same after you have had your baby. Accept offers of help gratefully and channel them usefully to enable you to enjoy the new life you have brought into being.

PREPARING THE BABY'S ROOM

Space may dictate whether or not your baby has its own room or whether he or she will be in with you. There are advantages and disadvantage to both arrangements.

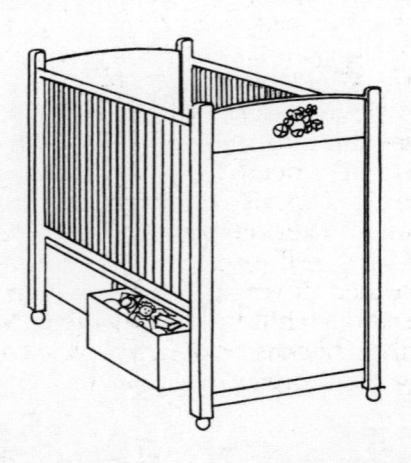

ADVANTAGES OF BABY BEING IN YOUR ROOM

☆ Near for you to attend to needs in the night.
☆ You only have to heat one room.
☆ You can hear the crying immediately.
☆ Feeling of closeness.

DISADVANTAGES

☆ You will wake for every snuffle, grunt and so on, and babies make a lot of these.
☆ If you intend the baby to stay with you for only a short while then she will have to re-adjust to another room.
☆ May inhibit re-establishment of sexual relationship.
☆ May disturb partner at night when you get up to feed her — perhaps this is an advantage!

It is certainly **not** essential that the baby has a room to herself. If you have older children a baby may disturb them during the night, although, like your partner, they soon acclimatize! Perhaps you can make one corner of your room into the baby's area by using a screen or wardrobe. If you use a lamp with a low watt bulb you will be able to see adequately.

If you are planning a room especially for the baby the most important thing to remember is that it should be flexible. Children's needs vary and change rapidly during the early years. If you intend the room to be used for playing in later on, paint will become scratched and decor will be 'well used', so choose things that can be easily renovated. If you are relaxed about the use of the room then your child will enjoy being in it.

The following checklist will help you to think about how to arrange and organize the room:

DISADVANTAGES

1. HEATING

Babies' rooms are often kept far too warm. The ideal temperature is 20°C/68°F at least for the first few weeks. If you do not have a thermostat on the radiators, you could buy a room thermometer. If you need to buy a heater, choose this with care from free–standing blower or convector heaters, electric or gas fires. Remember to fit a fire guard to all gas, oil or coal fires. All too soon your small baby will be on the move and accidents can and do happen. Gas and oil heaters need proper ventilation or they can be dangerous. Check them out with a qualified installer and have all equipment regularly serviced. Sometimes the room can feel very dry and a humidifier may help this.

2. WINDOWS

All windows should be fixed with safety catches and, if necessary, window bars so that she will be unable to fall out. The bars should be removable in case of fire. It is well worth draught–proofing windows. If you are making curtains, line them. Remember your baby will be going to bed earlier than you, and waking earlier. For daylight hours, you can buy special black-out lining from large department stores. Although this is expensive it may give you a few more lie-ins when the sun is rising early! Alternatively, you can use a blanket fixed to curtain rings. Blinds are another alternative.

3. FLOORS

The floor should be easy to clean because things will get spilt. If you have a family history of asthma or allergy, carpets are not a good idea as they trap dust and mites which can exacerbate the problem. Vinyl flooring is good, practical and fairly cheap. If you use rugs or mats,

DISADVANTAGES

make sure that you have anti-slip backing underneath or they will be dangerous.

4. FURNITURE

All previously painted furniture will need repainting with non-toxic lead-free nursery paint. Any wobbly furniture should be fixed to the wall so that it cannot topple onto your child when she pulls herself up to walk. You will probably need a chest of drawers, a wardrobe and a comfortable low chair and table for you to sit in while you feed. Most women, these days, use changing mats to change their baby on, and this is most safely done on the floor. If you use a changing mat on top surfaces never leave your baby unattended.

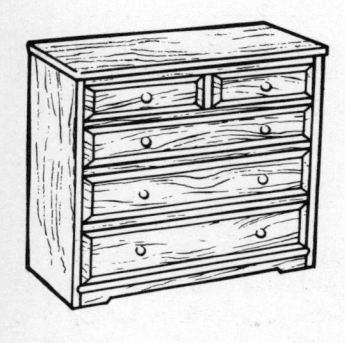

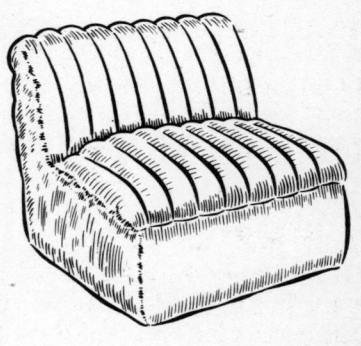

DISADVANTAGES

5. WALLS

Although wallpaper is lovely to look at it is less durable in a young child's room. It is easily marked with crayons, pulled off by inquisitive fingers and, unless it is washable, gets grubby-looking, particularly near the cot or changing area. Painted walls are much easier to clean. You can always make a frieze or stencil around it to brighten it up.

6. LIGHTING

It is best not to use lamps in a baby's bedroom as they can so easily be knocked over. Fix a dimmer switch to the central light so that you can creep in and check your baby without disturbing her. Make sure all electrical sockets are fitted with childproof covers. These are available from all good nursery stores.

7. SAFETY

Look at your home and think about what may need to be altered. A good way of finding out is by getting down physically to a child's height and wandering around to see what is accessible and what is potentially dangerous. Ask your health visitor for advice. Useful safety-first leaflets are available from Mothercare, Boots and Child Action Prevention Trust (see page 88).

FINISHING TOUCHES

Giving up work will put a strain on your finances so here are some ideas that you can make at home. None of them requires much skill, but it is nice to use things that you have made whilst 'in waiting'.

1. STENCILS

Stencils can be bought fairly cheaply from most decorating stores. You can use them to make a frieze or to brighten up odd bits of furniture in your baby's room. Look for pre-cut stencils because they are much easier to use, and make sure you buy quick-dry paint. Some stencils come in packs with brushes and paint and this is a good way to start. Stencils are also available from:

Stencil Decor: (they also supply paint crayons that do not smudge). Eurostudio Ltd, Unit 4, Southdown Industrial Estate, Harpenden, Herts AL5 1PW (0582 766001)

Carolyn Warrender: 91 Lower Sloane Street, London SW1W 8DA (071-730 0728). She has transparent plastic stencils which are easier to line up to see what you have done!

Lyn Le Grice Stencil Design Ltd: Bread Street, Penzance, Cornwall TR18 2EQ (0736 69881)

Full details of how to use stencils come on the packs.

FINISHING TOUCHES

2. WALLPAPER BORDERS

Many wallpaper companies make lovely nursery friezes which are either ready pasted or come with a peel–off backing. The border can be used at the top of the walls, at dado rail height (chair back level) or around the skirting board. You can also buy ready–made friezes which you can attach with adhesive tabs so that they can be removed easily for cleaning or when you are tired of them! Be imaginative in your use of stencils and borders. How about:

☆ Using stencils and fabric paints to stencil fabric for curtains, quilt covers or cushions.
☆ Paint an old chair in a bright colour and stencil the baby's name on it.

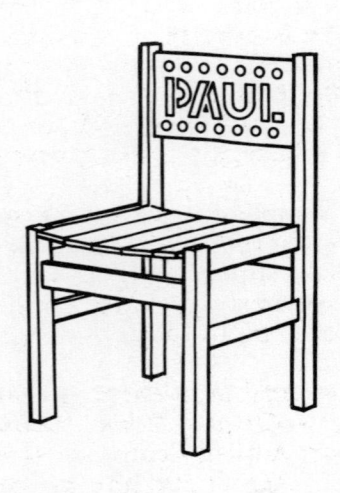

FINISHING TOUCHES

☆ Use stencils to brighten up a plain wood frame of a picture or to personalize a pin-board for your baby's room.

☆ Borders can be cut up and used individually on doors or furniture. Protect these with clear polyurethane varnish.

☆ Stencil the floorboards and then protect them with at least two layers of polyurethane varnish.

Are you artistic — or are your friends? Wall murals look wonderful and are a cheap way of making a room very special. Use an emulsion paint for quick drying. Small trial pots of paint are useful for adding tints to other colours or for highlighting faces, letters and numbers on the mural.

Mark up the wall you intend to use and measure it accurately. It can be easier if you draw out the design on graph paper and transfer it square-by-square onto the wall. At first transfer it using chalk, so that you can easily make alterations. Give yourself a few days to live with it before you paint it in. Some brilliant ideas seem less so a few days later!

Although it is tempting to start with small detailed bits, get the sky or top of the mural and any large spaces painted in first. Make sure each colour is completely dry before you paint the next area. Once finished the mural should be protected by two coats of eggshell varnish with a tint of blue.

A useful book to read in connection with murals and home decorating is *Creative Home Decorating* (Ward Lock). The Dulux Advice Centre at Wexham Road, Slough, Berks SL2 5DS will also give advice on painting problems.

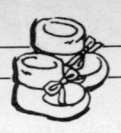

WHAT YOU NEED FOR YOUR BABY

Once you have established that you are pregnant, one of the first things you will find yourself doing is looking at other babies when you are out and about. Observing how other women are coping with their babies is one of the best ways of deciding what you will need for your baby.

The shops are full of tempting things to buy, but are they all necessary and what is essential? If you go to an ante-natal clinic you will have a chance to hear and talk about the sort of clothing that a new baby needs. But first it is important to think about your lifestyle.

1. Where do you live? In a house
   In a flat
   With parents
2. Do you have a garden or somewhere to dry clothes?
3. Do you have a washing machine?
4. Do you have a tumble–drier?
5. How far is the nearest launderette?

Question 1 will help you to think about space to store things. There is no point in buying things which are not needed immediately if you have no space to store them. Wait until nearer the time. When you think about where you live, look at the access to it. Are you far from the

WHAT YOU NEED FOR YOUR BABY

local shops and facilities? How easy is it to get to your front door? Do you live upstairs in a flat or maisonette? If the access to your home is difficult it may influence your decision as to whether to buy a pram, carrycot or buggy for transporting your baby. If you have a car, life may appear a little easier, but you will need to think about safety and how easily you can get the carrycot and other equipment in and out of the doors.

Questions 2, 3, 4 and 5 will help you to think about the practicalities of washing and drying your baby's clothes and bedding. Remember when you are buying baby clothes to look at the washing labels. Look for easy–care clothes that will dry easily and need little ironing, particularly if you have little space to dry things. Clothes that need handwashing may look lovely in the shops, but they do create extra work.

Think about when your baby will be born, and the sort of things that you usually like to do in that season. If you play a lot of tennis or other sports it may be that your baby will spend a lot of time in a carrycot or a pram near a tennis court. The amount of indoor and outdoor clothes that you buy will, to a certain extent, depend on your lifestyle and of course your purse. It is also important to think about the heating in your home. It is dangerous to overwrap and overheat babies, so if you have central heating you will need less thick jumpers and cardigans. Warm, light bedding is preferable to several layers of clothes. If your baby is going to be transported a lot in a baby sling or pushchair during the winter months, then obviously you will need to think about warm, waterproof and windproof clothing.

Here is a checklist of essential items of clothing that you will need for your baby in the first three months:

☆ Two towels for baby's use only.
☆ Twenty-four nappies or disposable nappies.
☆ Six plastic pants and pins (if using terry nappies).

WHAT YOU NEED FOR YOUR BABY

☆ Three cot blankets (these can be folded double at first if necessary).
☆ Four cot sheets.
☆ Four baby all-in-one suits.
☆ One outdoor all-in-one depending on season.
☆ Shawl or blanket to wrap the baby in when feeding.
☆ Six vests.
☆ Pram sheets and or buggybag.
☆ Two matinée jackets or cardigans.
☆ Bonnet.
☆ Two pairs of mittens.
☆ Two pairs of bootees or socks.
☆ Three bibs.

Talk to other mothers about which clothes wash and wear well, and which other items, in their opinion, are useful. Do not buy too much for the first three months because you will probably get clothes as presents and your baby's birthweight is not yet known. Will it be 2.25 kg/ 5 lb or 5 kg/10 lb? If you have few clothes to begin with you will find out which are easiest to get on the baby, wash best and dry quickest. It might not be the ones you imagine.

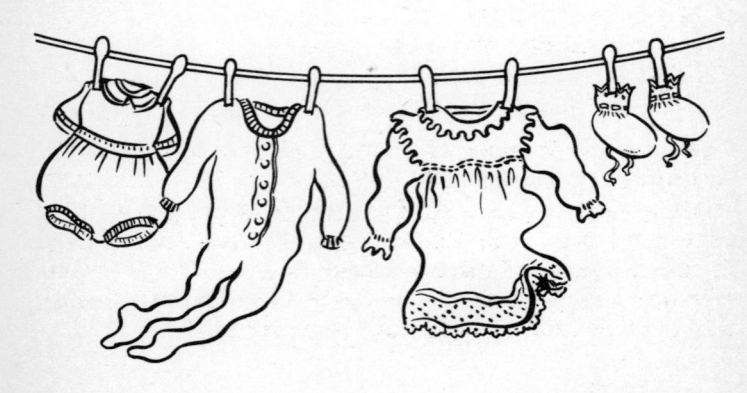

ESSENTIAL ITEMS OF EQUIPMENT

☆ Pram/carrycot or buggy with safety harness.
☆ Cot or crib and mattress.
☆ Nappy bucket and lid if using terry nappies.
☆ Baby relax chair.
☆ Baby sling.
☆ Baby bath.

If bottle–feeding.
☆ *Six feeding bottles and teats.*
☆ *Sterilizing unit and tablets or liquid.*

Of course, the amount and type of baby equipment that you buy will depend on your financial situation. Baby equipment is extremely expensive and the State Maternity Benefits will not go very far in providing it.

SOCIAL SECURITY BENEFITS

You will find the information you need in order to obtain the benefits that you are entitled to in the following leaflets:

☆ Maternity Benefits (N.I.17A)
☆ Babies and Benefits (FB8)
☆ Child Benefit (CH1)
☆ One parent Benefit (CH11)

These can be obtained from the leaflets unit, PO Box 21, Stanmore, Middlesex HA7 1AY.

Many post offices also have the leaflets. If you need advice to help you claim, contact your local Social Security Office or Citizens' Advice Bureau. The Maternity Alliance and National Council for One–Parent Families will also be able to help you. (See page 90.)

COMPLAINT PROCEDURE

Remember to keep all your receipts for clothing and equipment in case you need to take anything back or change it. Most shops are very good about changing faulty or defective equipment, but if you have problems or come across an item that you think is dangerous, contact your local Trading Standards Office.

BUYING SECOND-HAND

One way to reduce the cost of all the new equipment and clothing is to buy second-hand. Before you go ahead, however, there are a few points to bear in mind.

1. Is the item safe? Many items made as recently as five years ago were not covered by BSI standards.
2. If the item is painted or you intend to repaint it, make sure that you use special lead-free nursery paint.
3. Check cot mattresses thoroughly. The mattress should exactly fit the cot and leave no dangerous gaps. If it looks stained, or does not fit, or has a plastic covering, do not buy it.

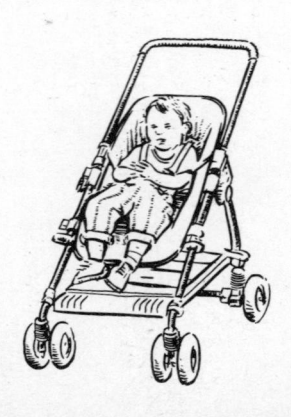

BUYING SECOND-HAND

4. Items bought second-hand will not have care or caution notices on them. Ask the shopkeeper or vendor if there are any particular things you should know.

5. When you buy a pram or buggy check that brakes, screws or harness points are all safe and secure. This rule applies to all baby transport items, even if you bought it new for a first baby and you are now going to use it for a second baby.

A very useful leaflet *Keep Your Baby Safe* with safe-buying tips is available from the Child Accident Prevention Trust. Please send a large SAE to CAPT, 28 Portland Place, London W1N 4DE.

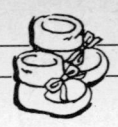

MUM'S ESSENTIALS

Some women are so thrilled to be pregnant that they want the world to know immediately and go out at once to buy smock-type dresses and 'maternity' styles. That is a very natural reaction, but remember that pregnancy lasts nine months and the seasons will change. The more normal time to change to maternity clothes is by about 12 weeks of pregnancy when ordinary clothes, such as trousers and skirts, become a bit uncomfortable as the uterus enlarges out of the pelvis.

Try to choose different colours and styles to cheer you up. It is amazing what a new lipstick or piece of jewellery will do, too, to perk you up. With luck, your hair will look more lustrous during pregnancy, although pregnancy is not a good time to have a perm. Talk to your hairdresser about a change of style.

So what do you need to think about when choosing clothes to wear throughout pregnancy? Unless you are made of money you will want to buy things that will still look good after many washes. Natural fabrics, such as wool and cotton, are more comfortable during pregnancy, because you will find that your body temperature is generally warmer in pregnancy because of increased blood circulation.

★ *UNDERWEAR* Your breasts will be one of the first things to change during the early weeks of pregnancy. If you have not previously worn a bra, you will

MUM'S ESSENTIALS

probably feel more comfortable with one. It is important to get a well-fitting bra, so ask to be measured properly. All good stores, stocking maternity wear, will be happy to help you. Cotton bras, though usually less fashionable looking, are often the most comfortable. Towards the end of your pregnancy, have your bra size checked again particularly if you are going to breast-feed. Cotton pants are also usually more comfortable than nylon ones. They are more absorbent and allow more air to circulate. This helps to prevent thrush. Bikini pants are more comfortable at the end of pregnancy.

★ *TIGHTS*

You can buy maternity tights from most big stores, but some women find tights too restricting during pregnancy. Support tights are particularly useful if your job entails a lot of standing about, or if you are suffering from varicose veins. Otherwise wear knee-high socks — there are so many good styles available now and if your skirt or dress is long enough, who will know!

★ *SHIRTS AND BLOUSES*

Usually it is only necessary to buy a size larger (or borrow some of your partner's). If you are going to breast-feed, check that any you do buy open easily down the front.

MUM'S ESSENTIALS

★ **TROUSERS AND SKIRTS**
Often you wear ordinary elasticated waist skirts and trousers well into pregnancy, especially if you wear a shirt or jumper over the waistband. What waist? Never mind it will come back. You can buy maternity trousers which have an elasticated front gusset and these are especially useful in the winter. Track suits bought one size larger are also ideal and very comfortable.

★ **DRESSES**
The maternity smock comes in many different designs, so you do not need to look like a galleon in full sail all the time. Remember that it may be a few months after the birth before you can get back into non-maternity clothes, so if you intend to breast-feed a couple of maternity dresses that open down the front will be helpful. If you can sew, there are maternity sections in the pattern books which give a range of different styles for you to make.

★ **JUMPERS AND CARDIGANS**
Again, you can raid your partner's wardrobe if he is bigger than you. Otherwise look out for nice baggy jumpers and buy a large size. Remember to buy long–line ones to allow for the bump. Cardigans are extremely useful because they keep you warm and don't always need to be done up. They are ideal, too, if you are breast-feeding.

MUM'S ESSENTIALS

★ SHOES

Although high-fashion shoes may be tempting, it is best to wear low- or flat-heeled shoes during pregnancy. Brighten them up with removable shoe bows when you go out. Shoes worn in pregnancy often do not fit afterwards, because during pregnancy your feet may swell and you will tend to walk slightly differently. This changes the shape of the shoes and makes them unsuitable for your non-pregnant use.

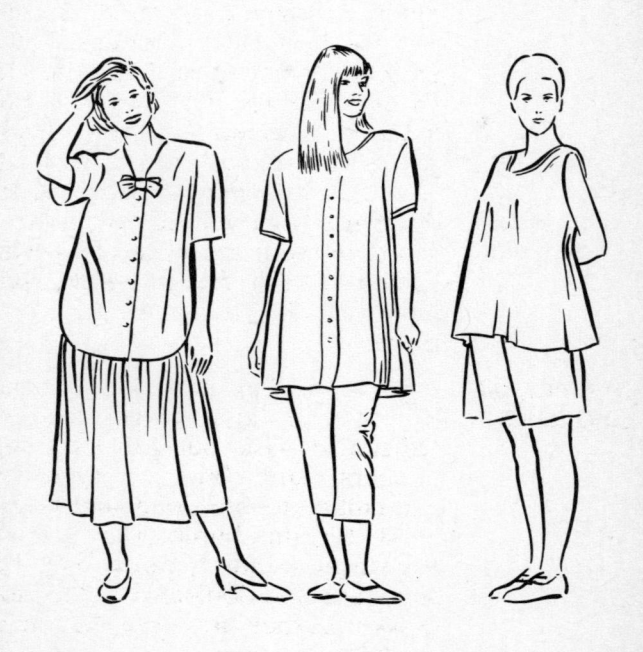

GETTING READY FOR BIRTH

If you are going to have your baby in hospital, the hospital will probably give you a list of items to bring in with you. You need to remember that there will not be much space to put anything. Whoever accompanies you to the hospital may well be asked to take your outdoor clothes and bag home. So what are you going to need?

☆ Two or three nightdresses which are easy to wash and open down the front if you want to breast-feed.
☆ Dressing gown and slippers.
☆ Two or three bras. These should be special cotton nursing bras for feeding the baby.
☆ Sanitary towels — super–absorbent stick–ons are most comfortable.
☆ Comfortable cotton pants.
☆ Wash–bag with two different coloured flannels for top and bottom! Toothbrush, toothpaste, hairbrush, shampoo and soap.
☆ Tissues.
☆ Make–up.
☆ Coins for the hospital payphone and telephone numbers.

Also useful are:

☆ A good moisturizing cream (hospital wards are very warm and your skin may get very dry).
☆ Snacks, i.e. muesli bar, packets of raisins, small packs of biscuits (for in-between nibbles).
☆ Book to read.
☆ Writing paper or notecards.
☆ Personal stereo and tapes.
☆ Ear plugs.
☆ A rubber ring to sit on and a pillow case to cover it, in case you have stitches.

GETTING READY FOR BIRTH

It is also useful to know what other women have found useful:

☆ You may feel happier in a large T-shirt or nightie than a hospital gown.
☆ A cardigan and woolly socks in case you get chilly.
☆ Small games, cards, paper and pencil to while away the time.
☆ A frozen ice pack or hot–water bottle to ease backache.
☆ Sponge or flannel, or mineral water spray, to mop your face.
☆ Lip salve.
☆ Small cartons of fruit juice and glucose tablets. (Check with the midwife before drinking, though, that this is all right.)
☆ Camera and film.
☆ Food to sustain your partner!

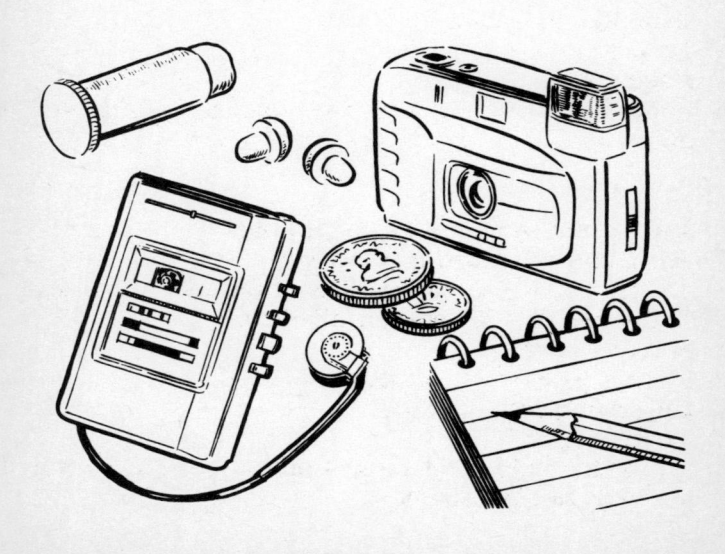

GETTING READY FOR BIRTH

It is also wise to pack a bag of clothes for your partner to bring in for you when you go home. This is usually easier than expecting one's partner to match up clothes, and saves arguments when you find there is only one shoe!

You will also need to bring things in for the baby. Again the hospital will probably have its own list but here are the essentials:

☆ Nappies and pins.
☆ Baby toiletries.
☆ Clothes to go home in.

Do not forget to fit a baby car seat or carrycot restraints in your car *before* you go in to hospital. Your baby's first ride home should be a safe one. Also leave a list of useful telephone numbers by the telephone for your partner, for example parents, hospital, close friends, and so on.

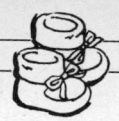

PREPARING FOR LABOUR

No doubt you will have heard many tales of labours since you announced that you were pregnant, but what you need to keep in mind is that, whatever you have heard, yours will be different because you are different!

Ante-natal classes certainly help to prepare both your mind and your body for labour, and this preparation will undoubtedly be of help. Fear of the unknown is far worse than going into something that you have thought about and planned.

WHAT IS LABOUR?

A hormone, oxytocin, will start labour off by causing the bands of muscle in your uterus (womb) to contract. You may feel these contractions very irregularly at first as a hardening of your abdomen together with a menstruation–type ache. The contractions will get closer and closer together, signifying established labour.

In this first stage of labour the muscles of the uterus are pushing the baby's head down. The longer muscles of the body of the uterus are also working to dilate the neck of the womb (cervix). Once the contractions are coming approximately every three minutes you should go into hospital. If the pain is difficult for you to control, or if your waters break (the fluid around the baby), you may feel you want to go into hospital immediately.

PREPARING FOR LABOUR

In the second stage of labour the cervix is fully dilated (open) and the muscles start to push the baby out into the vagina until it emerges.

The third stage of labour is when the placenta (afterbirth) is delivered and the labour is completed.

In many hospitals you will be asked if you have a 'birth plan'. This is a description of how, if everything is going well, you would like your labour to be managed. A very helpful discussion of birth plans can be found in *Freedom and Choice in Childbirth*, by Sheila Kitzinger, published by Viking. You can include on this how you feel about Caesarean section, episiotomy (See 8 below) and the delivery of the placenta (See 11 below). Although the birth plan is not legally binding it will act as a guide for the midwife to respect your wishes. You have every right to change your mind, of course, and the midwife and obstetrician will also give you advice on what action they feel is appropriate. It is helpful if you have discussed your ideas with your partner beforehand, so that he is able to support you in making decisions during labour.

SUGGESTIONS FOR YOUR BIRTH PLAN

1. Can my partner be with me all the time?
2. Once in labour can I walk around or must I stay in bed?
3. What about monitoring the baby — does it happen continuously? — Can I choose?
4. Are different birth positions encouraged, for example, squatting, using a birthing chair, water births, etc.?
5. Will I have to be shaved, have an enema or suppositories?
6. Will the membranes be ruptured (some hospitals routinely break the waters if labour does not progress)?
7. Are you willing to have the birth induced (speeding

SUGGESTIONS FOR YOUR BIRTH PLAN

up labour with a drip or pessaries)?
8. Episiotomy — an incision that is done routinely in some hospitals to help the baby out. Good midwifery support, however, often allows a woman to deliver her baby without an episiotomy.
9. Pain relief: Entonox (gas and air)
    Pethidine injection
    Epidural
    Natural birth.
10. How do you want to receive your baby, for example, instantly onto your tummy; wrapped and into your arms; breast-fed immediately.
11. Delivery of the placenta. An injection is usually given as the baby is delivered to help the uterus to contract and stop the risk of extra bleeding. Some women, however, prefer not to have this injection because they do not want the hormone passed on to the baby. You can ask not to have it, but be guided by the midwife.

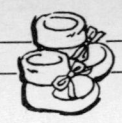

USEFUL ORGANIZATIONS AND FURTHER INFORMATION

Action on Smoking and Health (ASH)
5–11 Mortimer Street,
London W1N 7RH 071–637 9843)

Alcohol Concern
305 Gray's Inn Road,
London SW1X 8QF
(071–833 3471)

Association for Improvements in the Maternity Services (AIMS)
163 Liverpool Road,
London N1 0RF

Association for Post-Natal Illness
7 Gowan Avenue,
London SW6 6RH (071–731 4867)

Association for Breast-Feeding Mothers
131 Mayow Road,
Sydenham,
London SE26 4HZ (081–778 4769)

Association for Radical Midwives
62 Greetby Hill,
Ormskirk,
Lancashire L39 2DT (0695–72776)

British Diabetic Association
10 Queen Anne Street,
London W1M 0BD (071–323 1531)

British Homoeopathic Association
27a Devonshire Street,
London W1N 1RJ (071–935 2163)

Caesarean Support Network
2 Hurst Park Drive,
Huyton,
Liverpool L36 1TF

Child Accident Prevention Trust
28 Portland Place,
London W1N 4DE

Council for Complementary and Alternative Medicine
19a Cavendish Square,
London W1M 9AD (071–409 1440)

USEFUL ORGANIZATIONS

Foresight
The Old Vicarage,
Church Lane,
Witley,
Godalming,
Surrey GU8 5PN

Gingerbread
35 Wellington Street,
London WC2E 7BN
(071–240 0953)

Independent Midwives'
Association
65 Mount Nod Road,
Streatham,
London SW16 2LP

Institute for Complementary
Medicine
21 Portland Place,
London W1N 3AF (071–636 9543)

International Centre for Active
Birth
55 Dartmouth Park Road,
London NW5 1SL (071–267 3006)

La Leche League
BM 3424
London WC1N 3XX
(071–242 1278)

Maternity Alliance
15 Britannia Street,
London WC1X 9JP (071–837 1265)

National Association for the
Childless
318 Summer Lane,
Birmingham B19 3RL

National Childbirth Trust
Alexandra House,
Oldham Terrace,
London W3 6NH (081–992 8637)

USEFUL ORGANIZATIONS

National Council for One-Parent Families
255 Kentish Town Road,
London NW5 2LX (071-267 1361)

National Information for Parents of Prematures: Education, Resources and Support (NIPPERS)
49 Allison Road,
Acton,
London W3 6HZ (081-992 9310)

Relate (National Marriage Guidance Council)
Herbert Gray College,
Little Church Street,
Rugby CV21 3AP (0788 73241)

Pre-Eclampsia Toxaemia Society (PETS)
Eton Lodge,
8 Southend Road,
Hockley,
Essex SS5 4QQ (0702 205088)

Sickle Cell Society
Green Lodge,
Barretts Green Road,
Park Royal,
London NW10 7AP (081-961 7795)

Society to Support Home Confinements
Lydgate,
Lydgate Lane,
Walsingham,
Bishop Auckland DL13 3JA
(0388 528044 after 6 pm)

Standing Conference on Drug Abuse (SCODA)
1-4 Hatton Place,
Hatton Garden,
London EC1N 8ND
(071-430 2341)

Thalassaemia Society United Kingdom
107 Nightingale Lane,
London N8 7QY (081-348 0437)

Twins and Multiple Births Association
c/o Mrs Jenny Smith,
41 Fortuna Way,
Aylesby Park,
Grimsby,
South Humberside DN37 9SJ

Vegan Society
33-35 George Street,
Oxford OX1 2AY (0865 722166)

Vegetarian Society of the UK
Parkdale,
Dunham Road,
Altrincham,
Cheshire WA14 4QG

West London Birth Centre
33 Colebrooke Avenue,
London W13 8JZ

Women's Health and Reproductive Rights Information Centre
52 Featherstone Street,
London EC1Y 8RT
(071-251 6580/6332)

SUPPORT AND HELP IF YOU LOSE YOUR BABY

Foundation for the study of Infant Deaths (Cot Death Research and Support)
15 Belgrave Square,
London SW1X 8PS
(01–235 1721/0965)

Miscarriage Association
18 Stoneybrook Close,
West Bretton,
Wakefield,
West Yorkshire (0924 85515)

Stillbirth and Neonatal Death Society (SANDS)
28 Portland Place,
London W1N 3DE (01–436 5881)

Support After Termination for Abnormality (SATFA)
29–30 Soho Square,
London W1V 6JB (01–439 6124)

USEFUL MAGAZINES

All the parent magazines carry articles on Pregnancy.
Try: *Practical Parenting*
   Mother
   Mother and Baby
   Parents

USEFUL BOOKS

Active Birth: Janet Balaskas; Unwin 1983
When Pregnancy Fails: Judith Borg & Susan Lasker; Routledge & Kegan Paul
Exercises For Childbirth: Barbara Dale & Johanna Roeber; Century 1982
Yoga & Pregnancy: Sophy Hoare; Unwin 1985
Birth at Home: Sheila Kitzinger; OUP
All About Twins: Gillian Leigh; Routledge & Kegan Paul
You — After Childbirth: J. McKenna, M. Polden, M. Williams; Churchill Livingstone
The Home Birth Handbook: Monaco & Junor; The Manor House, Thelnetham, nr. Diss, Norfolk

SUPPORT AND HELP IF YOU LOSE YOUR BABY

From Here To Maternity: Anne Oakley; Penguin
Your Body, Your Baby, Your Life: Angela Phillips; Pandora Press
Pregnancy: Free from your local clinic or GP.
The Complete Mothercare Manual: Conran Octopus.
Mothercare Pregnancy Week by Week: Nina Grunfeld; Conran Octopus.

USEFUL VIDEOS

The Open University Courses: *Getting Ready for Pregnancy; Understanding Pregnancy and Birth;* Information from Centre for Continuing Education, The Open University, P.O. Box 188, Milton Keynes, MK3 6HW
Breast Feeding — If You Want To You Can: Available from video shops.

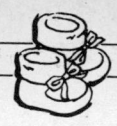

INDEX

Abnormalities, congenital, 42
Acupuncture, 39
Aerobics, 27
Alcohol, 10
Alcohol Concern, 10, 88
Amniotic fluid, 43, 44, 45
Ante-natal care, 85
   domino care, 20
   exercising, 26–8
   full hospital care, 20
   looking after your back, 28–9, 30, 32
   relaxation, 31
   shared care, 20
Ante-natal Clinics, 7, 8, 21–4
ASH (Action on Smoking and Health), 11, 88
Association for Breast-Feeding, 88
Association for Improvements in Maternity Services (AIMS), 88
Association for Post-Natal Illness, 88
Association for Radical Midwives, 88

Babies and Benefits leaflet (FB8), 75
Baby:
   development of, 40–6
   in your room, 65
   support and help if you lose, 91
   what you need for, 72–7
Baby clothes, 72, 73
   buying second-hand, 76–7
   essential items, 73–4
   washing and drying, 72, 73
Baby equipment:
   buying second-hand, 76–7
   essential items, 75
Baby Equipment Holder, 48–50
Baby's room, preparing, 64–71
   finishing touches, 69–71
   floors, 66–7
   furniture, 67
   heating, 66
   lighting, 68
   safety, 69
   windows, 66
Backache, 28–9, 30, 32
Bladder problems, 32
Bleeding in pregnancy, 13–14
Birth:
   getting ready for, 82–4
   home, 20–1
   hospital, 20, 21, 22
   inducing, 86–7
Birth plan, suggestions for, 86–7
Blood pressure, high, 11, 23
Blood tests, 23
Books and magazines, useful, 91–2
Bottle-feeding equipment, 75
Braxton Hicks contractions, 33
Breasts:
   doctor's examination of, 23
   fullness and sensitivity of, 15
British Diabetic Association, 88
British Homoeopathic Association, 39, 88
Buying:
   baby clothes and equipment, 73–5
   complaints procedure, 76
   maternity clothes, 78
   second-hand, 76–7

Caesarean section, 21, 86
Caesarean Support Network, 88
Cervix, 'incompetent', 13
Changing Bag, 51–2
Child Accident Prevention Trust, 77, 88
Child Benefit (CH1), 75
Chiropody, free, 25
Chiropractice, 39
Community Health Council, 24
Complaints procedure, 76
Conception, 8, 9, 12, 40

INDEX

Constipation, 15, 28, 30, 33, 37
Contractions, labour, 85
Co-op card, 23
Cot Death Research and Support, 91
Cot mattresses, second-hand, 76
Council for Complementary and
    Alternative Medicine, 88
Cystic fibrosis, 12
Cystitis, 33

Dental treatment, free, 25
Diabetes, 11, 23, 34
Diet, 9, 30, 36
Domino care, 20
Down's syndrome, 12
Drugs, drug-dependency, 11
Dungarees, 53–8

EDD (estimated date of delivery), 17
Entonox (gas and air), 87
Epidural, 7, 21, 87
Episiotomy, 7, 86, 87
Exercise, ante-natal, 26–8, 32
    classes, 28
    safety of, 28

Fainting, 34
Family Planning Clinics, 12, 15
Floors of baby's room, 66–7
Foetus *see* Baby, development of
Folic acid, 9
Foresight, 89
Freeline Social Security, 25
Furniture for baby's room, 67

Gas and air, 21, 87
Genetic counsellors, 12
Gingerbread, 89
GPs, 8, 12, 15, 17, 20

Headaches, 35
Health visitors, 8, 28
Heating of baby's room, 66
HIV (AIDS), 23
Home birth/delivery, 20–1
Homoeopathic remedies, 39
Hospital:
    ante-natal care, 20
    Ante-natal Clinics, 21–4
    birth of baby, 20, 21, 22
    crèche facilities, 25
    getting ready for birth in, 82–4
    preparing for labour, 85–7

Implantation bleed, 13
Independent Midwives' Association, 89

Indigestion, 28, 35
Incontinence, 28, 33
Institute for Complementary Medicine, 89
International Centre for Active Birth, 89

Knits for baby, 58–62
    cap, 61–2
    sweater, 58–60
    trousers, 60–1

Labour, 21
    artificially induced, 7
    pain relief during, 21
    preparing for, 85–7
    what is labour?, 85–6
Labour wards, 7
La Leche League, 89
Lighting (of baby's room), 68

Male fertility affected by alcohol, 10
Malnutrition, 9
Maternity clothes, 78–81
    dresses, 80
    jumpers and cardigans, 80
    shirts and blouses, 79
    shoes, 81
    tights, 79
    trousers and skirts, 80
    underwear, 78–9
Maternity Alliance, 25, 89
Maternity Benefits, 24–5, 75
Medicine and pills, 11, 39
    alternative, 39
Midwives, 7, 8, 22
    Community, 20
    Independent, 21
    Practice, 20
Miscarriage Association, 13, 91
Miscarriages, 13, 18, 28, 91
Monitoring the baby, 7, 86
Morning sickness, 15, 36
Moses Bag, 50
Mother-and-baby clubs, 24
Multivitamins, 9

National Association for the Childless, 12, 89
National Childbirth Trust, 7, 24, 28, 89
National Council for One Parent Families, 90
National Information for Parents of
    Prematures, 90
National Marriage Guidance Council, 90
Natural birth, 87
Nausea, sickness, 36

INDEX

One Parent Benefit (CH11), 75
Organizations, useful, 88–91
Overweight women, 9
Oxytocin, 85

Pain relief (in labour), 87
Parenthood groups, 8
Patchwork Blanket, 47–8
Periods, working out EDD from chart, 15, 16, 17
Pethidine, 21, 87
Piles (haemorrhoids), 28, 30, 37
Placenta (afterbirth), delivery of, 86, 87
Preconception, 8–9
Pre-Eclampsia Toxaemia Society, 90
Pregnancy, 7, 13–14
   ante-natal clinics, 21–4
   bleeding in early, 13–14
   confirmation of, 20–5
   development of baby, 40–6
   domino care, 20
   exercising, 26–8
   finding out about, 18
   full hospital care, 20
   hospital tests, 22–3
   miscarriage in, 13
   notebook, 19
   problems, 30–9
   relaxation, 31
   signs of, 15–17
Pregnancy tests, 15, 17
   do-it-yourself kits, 17
Progesterone, 32, 33, 35, 40

Relaxation, 31

Safety, 68, 77
SAFTA (Support After Termination for Abnormality), 91
SANDS (Stillbirth and Neonatal Death Society), 91
Sciatica, 32
SCODA (Standing Conference on Drug Abuse), 11, 90
Sewing designs for baby, 47–58
Shirodkar suture or stitch, 13
Sickle Cell Society, 90
Sleeplessness, 28, 38
Smoking, 10–11
Social Workers, 24
Social Security Benefits, 75
Society to Support Home Confinements, 90
Spina bifida, 9
Stencils, 69, 70–1
Swelling in pregnancy, 38
Swimming, 11, 32–3

Thalassaemia Society United Kingdom, 90
Thrush, 34
Tiredness in early pregnancy, 39
Trading Standards Office, 76
Trichomonas, 34
Twins and Multiple Births Association, 90

Ultrasound scans, 7, 8, 43
Urine, testing of, 23, 33

Vaginal discharge, 15, 34
Varicose veins, 37
Vegan Society, 90
Vegetarian Society of the UK, 90
Vernix, 45, 46
Videos, useful, 92

Wall murals, 71
Wallpaper borders, 70
Walls of baby's room, 68
Washing and drying clothes, 72, 73
West London Birth Centre, 90
Windows of baby's room, 66
Women's Health and Reproductive Rights Information Centre, 90
Work, at, 12

THE FAMILY MATTERS SERIES

Anniversary Celebrations 0 7063 6636 0
Baby's First Year 0 7063 6778 2
Baby's Names and Star Signs 0 7063 6801 0
Baby's Names 0 7063 6542 9
Barbecue Hints and Tips 0 7063 6893 2
Card Games 0 7063 6635 2
Card Games for One 0 7063 6747 2
Card Games for Two 0 7063 6907 6
Card and Conjuring Tricks 0 7063 6811 8
Charades and Party Games 0 7063 6637 9
Children's Party Games 0 7063 6611 5
Common Ailments Cured Naturally 0 7063 6895 9
Dreams and Their Meaning 0 7063 6802 9
Early Learning Games 0 7063 6771 5
Handwriting Secrets Revealed 0 7063 6841 X
How to be the Best Man 0 7063 6748 0
Microwave Tips and Timings 0 7063 6812 6
Modern Etiquette 0 7063 6641 7
Palmistry 0 7063 6894 0
Pressure Cooker Tips and Timings 0 7063 6908 4
Successful Children's Parties 0 7063 6843 6
Travel Games 0 7063 6643 3
Wedding Etiquette 0 7063 6868 1
The Wedding Planner 0 7063 6867 3
Wedding Speeches and Toasts 0 7063 6642 5